the handbook of Prescription Drugs

by Richard Burack, M.D.

the handbook of Prescription Drugs *Official Names, Prices, and Sources for Patient and Doctor*

PANTHEON BOOKS *A Division of Random House, New York*

Published in New York by Pantheon Books, a division of Random House, Inc.,
and simultaneously in Toronto, Canada, by Random House of Canada Limited.
Manufactured in the United States of America

Foreword

John Jones, a ten-year-old boy, was out of school for the greater part of the year. He had developed a sore throat and his parents had not sent him to see a physician. Two weeks later, he had become ill with joint pains and swelling, a fever and a fast pulse. He was found to have rheumatic fever; his heart had become involved.

With proper treatment, including penicillin, aspirin, and rest, John recovered. He was wisely ordered by his doctor to take a penicillin tablet every morning when he brushes his teeth and every night when he goes to bed and to do so until he is thirty or older. If John is faithful to this regimen, he will probably never have another attack of rheumatic fever, avoiding any further rheumatic damage to his heart.

John's parents and later John himself will have to buy a lot of penicillin—approximately 750 tablets a year. In twenty years he will have had to buy nearly 15,000 tablets. John's doctor might write either of the following prescriptions:

(A) ℞: John Jones
Pentids Tablets 200,000 units
Dispense 250
Sig: Label.[1] Take one twice daily on rising and at bedtime.

John Doe, M.D.

(B) ℞: John Jones
Potassium Penicillin G Tablets 200,000 units
Dispense 250
Sig: Label. Take one twice daily on rising and at bedtime.

John Doe, M.D.

Prescription A will cost about $27.50 at most drugstores. However, prescription B need cost only about $6.25, sometimes as little as $5.[2] Over twenty years A would cost $1650 and B $375.

Mrs. Mary Brown, thirty-five, suffers from seasonal asthmatic attacks. One morning in the late summer she woke up with the familiar wheeze and shortness of breath which in the past had always signified the start of three weeks of misery. This year Mrs. Brown's doctor decided that there was no contraindication to trying a short, three-week course of a steroid drug. The treatment was dramatically effective. The doctor might have written either of the following prescriptions:

[1] This is the common way to write prescriptions. Actually, it is redundant, for "Sig." (standing for the vocative "Signa") literally means "Label!" But, this is the traditional form.

[2] Prescription Drug List, Section I, "Drugs Used in Infectious Disease," page 84.

(A) ℞: Mary Brown
Meticorten 5 mgm
Dispense 100 tablets
Sig: Label. Take according to special daily dosage schedule as directed.

(B) ℞: Mary Brown
Prednisone 5 mgm
Dispense 100 tablets
Sig: Label. Take according to special daily dosage schedule as directed.

Prescription A would have cost between $28 and $30. Prescription B could have cost as little as $3 at many drugstores.[3]

Municipal Hospital, a 1000-bed institution run at taxpayer expense, has need each year for approximately 36,000 doses of a commonly prescribed laxative. The hospital pharmacy purchases the medication by the brand name "Colace," and pays about $756 a year for the drug. However, the pharmacy could buy the same number of doses for about $250 if it ordered the medication from any of a number of companies who market it by its official (generic) name, dioctyl sodium sulfosuccinate.[4]

In order to bring hypothetical situations such as these and many others to the attention of doctors and patients, I undertook to write this handbook. Let it be understood that the *Handbook* is not meant to be an indiscriminate, destructive attack upon a key industry which has flourished in an atmosphere of competition and free enterprise. The contributions of the American drug industry have been many and it deserves our gratitude. But the industry is not for this reason sacrosanct. If its nonscientist decision makers are guilty of using tactics that take unfair advantage of doctors and their patients, the public

[3] *Ibid.*, Section XIV, "Adrenal Steroids," page 144.

[4] *Ibid.*, Section XIII, "Drugs for Gastrointestinal Disorders," page 142. Note that cost to the pharmacist is more than twice as high as cost to the hospital, which buys large quantities (viz., 12,000 doses at a time).

should know what these tactics are and should be armed with information that will permit legitimate self-defense. Surely the public ought to know that too often it pays too much for prescription drugs and that—working with its physicians—it can do something about it right now, without sacrificing quality. This book is an attempt to demonstrate exactly what can be done.

I have tried to describe some of the more important of the complex reasons for the present unsatisfactory situation, and suggest that a partial remedy will come only through the discontinuation of the common practice of relying upon brand names for identification of drugs. Facts and figures are presented to support the view that there exists for the doctor no scientific or practical justification for prescribing drugs by brand name, and for the patient surely no economic justification. For it is a truism that "brand name" equals "higher price" because of higher advertising overhead. Furthermore, buying by brand name does not always ensure maximum efficacy and safety.

In order to help both doctors and interested patients, the *Handbook* provides a list of basic drugs, giving the official identification of drugs commonly referred to by unofficial names, and stating their prices, comparing the cost from a variety of sources. The Appendixes comprise a list of drug companies accepted as approved bidders by the Defense Supply Agency of the United States government, and a partial list of distributors of generic drugs. In the Index, all drugs listed in the *Handbook* are cross-indexed under both their trade and their generic names.

All prices listed are as of the last half of 1966. The *Handbook* will be revised as needed so that eventual price changes and new information on drugs may be included. I sincerely believe that most physicians will be pleased to have this information at hand both in their offices and in hospitals. It is my hope that the public, too, will find the contents of the *Handbook* useful and interesting.

Many people have encouraged me. I am especially grateful to Dr. Otto Krayer, Emeritus Professor of Pharmacology at Harvard Medical School; Mr. Benjamin Gordon, Staff Economist for the United States Senate Select Committee on Small Business; Dr. Irene Till, Professor of Economics at Howard University, who was Staff Economist to the Kefauver Subcommittee, and Mrs. Paula McGuire of Pantheon Books, an able editor. Several practicing pharmacist friends who have asked to be anonymous gave invaluable help, and a number of physician colleagues and nondoctor friends made useful suggestions. I am particularly indebted to Dr. H. Jack Geiger, Professor of Preventive Medicine at Tufts University College of Medicine, and Dr. Paul R. Draskoczy, Associate in Pharmacology at Harvard Medical School. Much gratitude is due Mr. Morton Mintz of the staff of the *Washington Post* whose excellent book *The Therapeutic Nightmare* provided intellectual stimulation.

Responsibility for facts, opinions, and any deficiencies is my own. The views expressed are not necessarily those of any institution or organization of which I am a member.

The patience and dedication of my secretary, Miss Karen Kutrieb, has earned my sincere appreciation.

November, 1966 R. B.

Preface

Among handbooks this is an exception—exceptional in the scope of the information it provides, the multiplicity of audiences to which it is addressed, and the number of purposes it aims to serve. It is exceptional, too, in the background which brought it into being, for medicine in the 1960s is almost entirely a product of the twentieth century. Although its foundations of natural science and systematic observation go far back, it was not until the methods of physics, chemistry, and microbiology began to be applied directly to the study of disease that the current information explosion began. Since then, applicable knowledge has accumulated geometrically.

Similarly the physician's potential ability to modify, ameliorate, and even cure disease has grown at a dizzying rate. Weekly, daily, and even hourly, new understanding is being developed through research, and for this reason, an ever-increasing number of new therapeutic agents of ever-increasing power and specificity are appearing.

Any such rapid growth, no matter how desirable, is certain to create problems and unwanted side effects—especially if allowed to proceed at random without control. Abuses are bound to occur and the symbiosis between medicine and industry, the physician and the pharmaceutical manufacturer, which has carried both so far so fast, like any such arrangement in biology has always been potentially open to distortion into parasitism by either party.

Because of this rapid growth, the teaching of clinical pharmacology in many medical schools has become insufficient to prepare physicians to use with maximum effectiveness and safety the multitudinous potent agents currently available for the treatment of their patients. Further postgraduate study has been precluded by the pressures of patients' demands for more care, and the physician has, perforce, resorted to the convenience of proprietary drug names and reliance on advertising for professional information—advertising designed not unexpectedly to promote "positive thinking" about a product's possible uses rather than its potential side effects or dangers, let alone its cost in comparison to other perhaps equally effective agents. Not only is it obviously undesirable that the physician, by accepting advertising as a major information source, lose his position of informed leadership in the development and use of new drugs, but with many competing for the same market, products inevitably multiply for economic rather than purely scientific reasons and advertising increases in volume and cost—costs which inevitably get paid by the patient, not his doctor or the drug manufacturer.

That these issues would someday have to be faced by physicians, their patients, the drug industry, and perhaps the government has long been clear. Yet the excitement of palpable miracles and the promise of still more to come has made concern with costs seem frivolous and blinded public and professional eyes to practices which never would have been accepted with equanimity had the movement been less fraught with the hectic excitement of discovery.

The public hearings conducted by Senator Kefauver and his colleagues were the first step toward reform. They brought to public attention a number of these problems and, by pointing to undesirable practices and abuses, set the stage for the development of closer control at the governmental level. However, control at this level alone is not enough.

The mission of this *Handbook* is to bring about the next steps by calling attention to the continuing presence of some undesirable practices and pointing out that their control will depend ultimately on action by individual physicians. Effectively as this proposition is presented, the book would be only of passing interest were it to stop there. What distinguishes it from other such statements is that it offers concrete advice on *how* abuses can be controlled by placing everyday practical therapeutics back under the guidance of sound pharmacologic principles. The lower costs which can accrue from such action add an additional compelling reason for physicians to change their current practices. The fact that the *patient* as well as his physician is addressed is more than just a mechanism to force the hand of the reluctant practitioner. The era when medicine needed to hide its ignorance behind a wall of mysticism is long gone. It is high time that more patients and physicians become partners in the treatment of illness—a situation which can only develop if *both* are fully informed.

Thus the list of drugs in this book, for all its deceiving brevity, subserves many purposes. It suggests to the medical student a framework on which to build his knowledge of clinical pharmacology. It provides the practicing physician with a much-needed guide for simpler and more effective therapy. It offers the patient understanding of what his physician is about. Finally, it provides information about costs and suggestions for controlling them which are of potential use to all interested in seeing an end to unbridled escalation in the expense of medical care.

GEORGE NICHOLS, JR., M.D.
Clinical Professor of Medicine, Harvard Medical School
Director, Department of Medicine, Cambridge City Hospital

Contents

Introduction

The Extent of Drug Promotion

The United States has reason for looking upon its medical profession with pride, for its medical schools and teaching hospitals have succeeded well in training doctors to make correct diagnoses and to perform proper surgery. Our level of medical practice is the envy of many nations because our practicing physicians and surgeons have managed, for the most part, to stay abreast of new, important developments in diagnostic and surgical techniques. That they have been able to do so is a tribute to the profession itself, which has taken the lead in encouraging their continuing education through the use of books, journals, postgraduate courses, lectures, and hospital staff conferences.

The great pity—bordering on scandal—is that too much responsibility for keeping doctors informed of developments in pharmacology has been forfeited to pharmaceutical manufacturers who have succeeded, through advertising, in influencing practicing doctors to write prescriptions for which the patient pays a maximum price. The immensity of this advertising effort is best appreciated by considering that it costs the drug industry at least $600,000,000 annually. Since there are approximately 200,000 prescribing doctors, the drug companies are spending more than 3000 advertising dollars each year on each doctor! These figures are taken from a prepared statement before the Subcommittee on Intergovernmental Relations of the House Committee on Government Operations by Dr. James L. Goddard, Commissioner of the United States Food and Drug Administration, May 25, 1966.

Much of this advertising is misleading. According to Dr. Goddard, in 1965 "one third of the members of the Pharmaceutical Manufacturers Association had violated FDA agency regulations on fraudulent or misleading advertising." Clearly, a third and interested commercial party has inserted itself into the doctor-patient relationship, yet no clear warning voice has been raised against it from within the medical profession. As Dr. Goddard said, the American doctor is "frankly under siege."

Why should doctors, among the best trained of all professional cadres in this country, be susceptible to misleading advertising? As medical students were they not provided with adequate education about drugs? The answer is that the great majority have been given an excellent, modern laboratory and lecture course in pharmacology, but, with few exceptions, there has been little organized review or systematic presentation of such material after the student's second year of medical school. This is because those faculty members who teach pharmacology are only rarely practicing doctors (clinicians) as well as scientists. The scholarly, research-oriented pharmacologist has usually had little or no experience in the actual use in humans of the drugs which he knows so well in theory. He may have no interest in clinical medicine, and even if he does, he will probably not feel qualified to play a significant role in case discussions before members of the clinical faculty. Unfortunately, very few of the clinical faculty have much more than a superficial interest in pharmacology as such, for tradition has taught that the cornerstone of the best medical practice is learning to diagnose. It is commonplace to hear, "Drug therapy is easy; once the diagnosis has been made, all you have to do is look up the recommended drug and prescribe it." While this may once have been a useful view, rapid developments in pharmacology (not all of them beneficial) have rendered it obsolete and its persistence has led to an obvious result: the student ceases to continue to learn in depth about drugs, and while he receives first-rate instruction in pathological physiology, diagnosis, and surgical treatment, he frequently adopts sloppy habits with regard to the prescription of therapeutic agents.

This unhappy state of affairs is by no means unknown to responsible members of medical school faculties, and there have been moves here and there to institute courses dealing in pharmacology during the latter two years of medical school, the so-called "clinical" years. For the practicing doctor, similarly, there is no coherent plan for periodically updating his knowledge of drugs and their use. Into the breach has stepped the pharmaceutical industry to persuade, to cajole, and to "educate." To be sure, there is now available to all doctors and medical students a biweekly loose-leaf sheet called *The Medical Letter*, published by Drug and Therapeutic Information, Inc., a nonprofit organization which fearlessly dispenses objective criticism of drugs old and new, but it is not meant primarily to give comprehensive information on prices. Simply written and intelligently critical, *The Medical Letter* deserves the fuller support of the profession, for the struggle to control doctors' habits of therapeutic practice is a big stake and the giant pharmaceutical corporations can be expected to continue to promote, advertise, and "educate" at an increasing rate, one which even now far exceeds in cost the combined administrative and teaching budgets of all the nation's medical schools put together.[1]

What is wrong with the adoption by pharmaceutical manufacturers of the role of educator of physicians about developments in drug therapy? Let us look first at some of the unfortunate prescribing practices encouraged by the advertising and promotion policies of these manufacturers, policies disclosed during the Kefauver hearings on drugs during the years 1960 to 1962.

1. Prescribing too many drugs too often. Many patients require no prescription, just an attentive listener, a careful examination by the doctor, and some reassurance. Too often there is a tendency to prescribe for these patients a sedative ("tranquilizer"), a vitamin capsule, thyroid or female hormones, an injection of vitamin B_{12} or penicillin, or some new drug X which the patient specifically requests. The unnecessary prescription of drugs is one of the hallmarks of second-rate medical practice, and yet when it occurs, the fault is not always entirely the doctor's. In the background there is often the fine hand of the pharmaceutical advertiser who makes an intense effort to reach the doctor through the patient. A physician, formerly of the medical staff of one of the best known and largest of the drug houses, testified before the Kefauver Subcommittee: "It is an unfunny joke in the medical profession that the very latest information on new advances in medicine most often appears in the eminent medical journals such as Reader's Digest, Time, and The Wall Street Journal. Some of this is legitimate good reporting. However, much of what appears has in essence been placed by the public relations staffs of the pharmaceutical firms. A steady stream of

[1] P.R. Garai, "The Pill the Doctor Must Swallow," *The Johns Hopkins Magazine*, Vol. XV, No. 7 (May 1964), pp. 7–9, 21–23.

magazine and newspaper articles are prepared for distribution to the lay press. These may take the form of so-called informative or background articles on conditions such as allergies or edema. Buried within the article, there is often a brief paragraph mentioning that a great drug has been discovered and manufactured by company X, and the name of the drug is given. The article does not say that the reader should rush to his physician and demand the drug, but the implication is usually clear. And, of course, there is nothing to show where the article originated."[2]

Small-town newspapers and lesser known periodicals are especially likely to carry information prepared by public relations experts. The larger daily newspapers and the major wire services have highly skilled science reporters who weed out most of the misleading or exaggerated public-relations drug claims and file them in their wastebaskets. In spite of this, much misinformation—particularly via small newspapers and some national magazines—does reach the public. One public relations executive interviewed by the Kefauver Subcommittee read from a letter sent by his own organization to a large drug company which was a prospective customer: "a news story on clinical results from a new drug or on the research achievements that went into this discovery automatically helps create a demand for the product." The letter, soliciting the patronage of the corporation, described what "in our opinion would have the broadest and most direct sales promotion results." This was a "feature column service providing health and medical stories built around some product for smalltown daily or weekly newspapers. Both text and illustrations are supplied in matrix form requiring no composition or engraving by the newspaper." The feature was reportedly sent to 2000 small papers, many of which could afford

[2] United States Senate, Committee on the Judiciary, Subcommittee on Antitrust and Monoply, 86th Congress, 2nd Session, *Hearings on S. Res. 238*, Part 18, pp. 10241 *et seq.*

no wire services and welcomed the availability of this free material. In the feature mat the name of a product was always mentioned. The public relations executive denied that his service was advertising in the strict sense and maintained, therefore, that the material need not be identified as such when published.[3]

According to another witness before the Subcommittee, a physician who had previously been chief medical director of another of the pharmaceutical giants: "The patients contribute their share [to the unnecessary prescription of drugs]. Too many are unable to accept that the physician . . . is still best able to determine the proper treatment. The best doctor is not necessarily the one who gives a shot for every complaint, and the more conservative physician who does not prescribe the latest drug reported in Coronet may be far more competent than the one who does. . . . To the pharmaceutical industry this is an open invitation to exploit both the patient and the doctor. . . ."[4]

2. Prescribing costly drugs of unproved clinical value. One good example is the long-acting blood-vessel dilator, usually an organic nitrate (not nitroglycerin), which is alleged to cause improvement in angina pectoris. There is evidence in the medical literature as convincing of the ineffectiveness of this class of compounds as of their effectiveness. When this is the case with any drug, a reasonable inference is that its usefulness is open to serious question; effective drugs usually give obvious results.

The so-called "tranquilizers" fall into this category, too. "The simple fact that anxiety is virtually impossible to evaluate objectively and that it responds to almost any bag of asafetida[5] accounts for the market in the so-called tranquilizers," according

[3] United States Senate, Committee on the Judiciary, Subcommittee on Antitrust and Monoply, 87th Congress, 2nd Session, *Hearings on S. 1552*, Part 6, pp. 3212 *et seq.*

[4] *Hearings on S. Res. 238*, Part 18, p. 10374.

[5] It was a common practice in the Middle Ages to wear suspended from the neck a cloth bag filled with asafetida, a foul-smelling weed, which was believed to ward off plagues, but in fact has no such action.

to the same ex-chief medical director of a large drug house who has already been quoted.[6] However, these agents can certainly be effective as placebos,[7] or, as mild sedatives, neither more nor less effective than small doses of phenobarbital. The point the *Handbook* wishes to make, therefore, is not that the practicing doctor should never under any circumstances prescribe them, but that if he does he should know how much his patient is forced to pay for them. He needs a source to tell him how to prescribe such a drug in its least expensive dose form and by its least expensive name.

3. Prescribing drugs with serious toxic side effects when there are equally effective, less toxic agents available. One example: though chloramphenicol is an effective drug and the agent of choice for treatment of certain rare infections (e.g. typhoid fever), its capacity to interfere with the ability of bone marrow to manufacture blood cells has been well known for years. Although this unwanted side effect most often occurs when more than the usual dose is given, there are rare persons in whom even a small dose can cause serious disease or even death. The argument that death from this cause is rare is no consolation to the families of the many persons who have been killed by unnecessary prescription of chloramphenicol. As long ago as 1952 the Food and Drug Administration required (upon the recommendation of the National Research Council) that chloramphenicol's package label and advertising carry the warning that it not be used indiscriminately or for minor infections, but its casual use persists. Again, it is not all the doctor's fault; the reader is referred to *Hearings on S. Res. 238*, Part 26, pp. 15945–15981, which contains documentary evidence showing that a manufacturer, with careful use of words, can manage to dilute the impact which a required

[6] *Hearings on S. Res. 238*, Part 18, p. 10374.

[7] A placebo is an inactive medication, e.g. a sugar pill, whose beneficial effect on the patient is due entirely to psychological factors.

warning label is intended to have. See also Senate Report No. 448, "Administered Prices: Drugs" (pp. 192–98). For further discussion see below under "The Nature of Drug Promotion."

4. Prescribing powerful and potentially toxic drugs for minor conditions. The classic example is the thalidomide tragedy, which this country was fortunately spared. Mild anxiety hardly requires treatment with drugs and surely not in pregnancy. The lesson of the terrible thalidomide-induced defects in newborn babies seems to have been driven home to most doctors in that the prescribing of any drug at all during early pregnancy is now undertaken only after the most serious consideration by all responsible physicians. On the other hand, it remains common practice to prescribe for a simple stuffy nose a systemically taken tablet or capsule which does indeed help the nasal stuffiness, but can at the same time cause a rise in blood pressure and a pounding or irregular heartbeat. Yet inexpensive, safer nose drops are known to be just as effective, though perhaps slightly less convenient.

5. Prescribing drugs without knowledge of official identity, sources of manufacture, and cost. It is common knowledge to pharmacologists and well-trained physicians that 90 percent or more of adult patients who are not sick enough to require hospitalization can be treated effectively with one or more of a small number of basic drugs, and the list of all such basic drugs is in fact a short one. Because most of these drugs are available by their official (generic) names at a cost far lower than when prescribed by unofficial (brand) names, treatment can usually be simple and inexpensive. Unfortunately, the intensive and highly effective advertising and promotion campaigns conducted by pharmaceutical manufacturers have muddied the waters and confused the well-intentioned and otherwise well-informed practicing doctor into believing that there are more essential drugs on the market than is actually the case. Furthermore, because responsibility for publishing lists of available drugs and their sources has been forfeited by the medical profession itself to the manufacturers of brand-name drugs, the manufacturers have effectively kept practicing doctors uninformed about the many sources of inexpensive drugs of purity, quality, and potency sold by their generic names. It is for these reasons that treatment is too often both complicated and costly.

How can a doctor care properly for the "whole person" unless he understands the impact of disease upon his patient's pocketbook? Obviously, he cannot. And it is here, on the question of cost to the consumer, that the pharmaceutical company's adopted role of educator most flagrantly breaks down, for there is in it an inherent self-interest which cannot be disguised.

In summary, then, far too often a patient takes a drug when he may need none at all. Or he takes a drug with dangerous side effects when a safer drug is available. Or he takes a drug of unproved clinical value, or one which carries important risks and therefore never should be given for minor conditions. In each of these situations—and even in the happy instance when the prescription is both justified and safe—the patient is far too likely to pay much more than is necessary.

Official and Unofficial Names of Drugs

The key to an understanding of why drugs often need not cost as much as they do is a knowledge of what is meant by the terms "official" and "unofficial" with respect to drug names.

New drugs and the processes by which they are made can be protected for seventeen years under United States Patent Law. Every new drug approved for sale must be given an official name (also called "generic"[8] or "nonproprietary"), and it is by this label that it is known to pharmacologists and to the medical students whom they teach. A new drug which is developed by a drug company is also endowed with an unofficial (also called "brand," "trade," or "proprietary") name, and this is the label by which the drug is advertised to the profession. Until only recently these advertisements were not even required to include a prominent display of the drug's generic name,[9] but now the law says that it must be included in letters at least one half as large as those used for the brand name. It is profoundly in the economic interest of the pharmaceutical manufacturer to "train" doctors and patients to use the brand name only, and the manufacturers have succeeded mightily in doing so. Approximately 90 percent of prescriptions in the mid-1960s are written using brand names.[10] Brand names are frequently easier to say, spell, and remember than generic names because it has been common for manufacturers to make the latter chemical tongue-twisters, which discourages their use. Besides, brand names have often been designed so as to imply what the pharmacological action of a drug is advertised to be, an effective merchandising technique: e.g., the officially named chlordiazepoxide, a sedative, is almost universally known as "Librium." Since 1961 generic names have been subject to approval by a committee, the United States Adopted Names Council (USAN), which includes representatives of the United States Pharmacopeial Convention, the American Pharmaceutical Association, and the American Medical

[8] Technically and correctly the term "generic" refers to classes or genera of drugs, but in common parlance it has come to be used interchangeably with "nonproprietary" and "official." To avoid confusion and pedantry, the *Handbook* adopts the popular usage.

[9] At one point during the Kefauver hearings the president of the Pharmaceutical Manufacturers Association, Dr. Austin Smith, found it impossible to locate the generic name on an advertisement until aided by a magnifying glass proffered by the Subcommittee counsel.

[10] *F-D-C Reports* ("*The Pink Sheet*"), Washington, September 5, 1966.

Association. Why "Adopted" rather than "Official"? And can any dignified official name compete with one designed to merchandise?

During the seventeen years that a patent is in effect, the original developer of the drug is free to take advantage of his privileged position to recoup his investment and reap the reward of profit for his risk and enterprise. After seventeen years, anyone else is free to help himself to the process described in the patent and to manufacture and market the drug on his own, *though he may not use the original brand name, which is limited by* trademark *law to the use of the original coiner.*

As an illustration, we can refer to the drug dextroamphetamine, widely used for its appetite-curbing properties. The substance was patented by Smith Kline & French Laboratories, who alone sold it in vast amounts for a seventeen-year period under the brand name Dexedrine. The patent has long since expired, and as of now, half a hundred companies are marketing dextroamphetamine, nearly all at lower prices than Smith Kline & French. But the many new producers of dextroamphetamine may not advertise it as Dexedrine. If Dexedrine is the word the doctor writes on the prescription blank by force of habit, the druggist must by law in thirty-nine states (except within institutions) dispense Dexedrine—and at its brand-name price. It must be pointed out, however, that even if the prescription read "dextroamphetamine," the druggist would be free to dispense Dexedrine at the higher price, and that is exactly what many of them do, since it is not yet common enough practice for drugstores to keep in stock the less expensive—but for practical purposes identical—dextroamphetamine tablets marketed by other companies without the trade name Dexedrine. Such less expensive, non-brand-name dextroamphetamine tablets are the "generic equivalents" of Dexedrine.

The Nature of Drug Promotion

Pharmaceutical companies influence doctors in several ways. For one thing, their salesmen, called "detail men," visit doctors' offices at frequent intervals to dispense samples, describe new products, remind the doctor of older ones, and sometimes to recite certain statements which the parent company considers of special importance and has ordered them to commit to memory. Many of these practices provide a service which the *Handbook* has no wish to denigrate. However, the major job of the detail man is to sell. Many doctors by now are aware that information obtained from the detail man must be examined critically, and that salesmen cannot be considered authoritative sources for continuing education about drugs. There is little chance to check on the accuracy of what the detail man tells the doctor in the privacy of his office, and there is plenty of opportunity for exaggeration, dissimulation, and outright concealment. During the course of the hearings on drugs conducted in 1960 by the Kefauver Subcommittee it was reported that the National Research Council recommended to the FDA that a label be placed on chloramphenicol (Parke, Davis's Chloromycetin®) warning that it should "not be used indiscriminately or for minor infections" because serious blood disease had occasionally been found to occur with its use. The report of the hearings contains a copy of a Parke, Davis President's Letter telling the firm's detail men of the new warning label but prefacing the announcement with the statement that "Chloromycetin has been officially cleared by the FDA and the National Research Council with *no restrictions* on the number or the range of diseases for which Chloromycetin may be administered." (Emphasis in original) Obviously, when the National Research Council recommended that chloramphenicol "not be used indiscriminately or for minor infections," it was proposing a restriction on the number and the range of diseases. The hearings report that in a Directors' Letter sent two months later to its detail men, Parke, Davis included "Planned Presentation 10," which contained arguments and figures designed to enable the detail man to allay apprehensions about the drug on the part of the physician. However, it is also reported that instructions accompanying the presentation carried this interesting admonition: "The special detail [Planned Presentation 10] should not be introduced unless the physician brings up the subject or unless you know that he has ceased prescribing Chloromycetin," a position hardly in keeping with the responsibility of drug manufacturers always to keep doctors fully informed on important matters.[11]

Thus, the detail man without realizing it himself can transmit information to doctors which is either misleading or false. In other cases he supplies misinformation for which the parent company cannot be blamed. As an example, a detail man recently tried to convince me that the United States Air Force had "three or four years ago" been "burnt" by the purchase of digoxin (the generic name for a commonly used heart drug) which turned out to be "only 47 percent of proper potency." It so happens that drugs used by the armed services are bought by generic name through secret bids and that all bidders must first pass inspection by the Defense Supply Agency; no delivery is accepted without check on identity, quality, purity, and potency of the material. It seemed, therefore, that either the detail man's story was incorrect or the Defense Supply Agency must have fallen down on the job. When I wrote to the man's company requesting more details, the vice president in charge of sales replied that the company was unaware of the incident. This points up the importance to the doctor of listening critically to the detail man. (For further discussion of this incident see pages 27–28.) Drug corporations are aware that detail men may, by accident or design, transmit

[11] United States Senate, Committee on the Judiciary, Subcommittee on Antitrust and Monopoly, 87th Congress, 1st Session, Senate Report No. 448, "Administered Prices: Drugs," pp. 192–96, and documentation in *Hearings on S. Res. 238*, Part 26, pp. 15945–81.

information which is not factual, and most guard against the possible repercussions of such practices by not supplying the men with stationery containing the company letterhead. Thus, misinformation is unlikely to be put in writing.

Advertisements in medical journals represent a second method of influencing the doctor's prescribing habits. Advertisement of drugs is entirely proper and can undoubtedly be useful to the medical profession. However, as mentioned earlier, advertisements are too often characterized by misrepresentation or misleading captions, in spite of the supervision of journal editorial boards and scrutiny by the Food and Drug Administration. Examples would fill a book.

The Kefauver hearings contain documentary evidence of an advertisement for a steroid drug with X-ray pictures of the large bowel showing typical changes seen in ulcerative colitis. Although the first picture was not labeled "before," the second was labeled "Barium enema following successful therapy for ulcerative colitis." One physician wrote the company (Upjohn) to question whether the X-rays were of the same patient. By the time correspondence between the company's advertising manager, its medical director, and the physician had come to an end, it was clear that these X-rays were from two different patients each with different degrees of ulcerative colitis, and that in fact neither one had ever been treated with a steroid. The company, denying intent to mislead, expressed regrets over the incident; its advertising agency refused to admit to any impropriety.[12] The prescribing of drugs is too serious and potentially dangerous to be influenced by less than factual objective material. And if some advertisements are misleading, how does the doctor know which ones to trust?

The deluge of "junk mail" which descends upon doctors daily is by now common knowledge, and most physicians are

[12] *Hearings on S. 1552*, Part 6, pp. 3084 *et seq.* and Part 7, pp. 3301–3310.

either too busy or too wise to pay it much attention. However, the cost of this material is passed on to the consumer. And few members of the medical profession are likely to be aware that their names are obtained for mailing lists through the offices of the American Medical Association, the source from which the advertisers buy their names and addresses. This is an important source of AMA revenue: according to the general counsel to the AMA, $900,000 of income was derived from this source in 1960.[13]

Probably the shrewdest and most effective means by which the big pharmaceutical corporations perpetuate their hold over doctor and patients is through the book *Physicians' Desk Reference* (*PDR*). Although some doctors may not think of it in these terms because its format and veneer give it a cleverly noncommercial, authoritative appearance, *PDR* is in fact composed of advertising. The 1966 rate is $115 per column inch. With more than 15,000 column inches, the gross value of space in the 1966 *PDR* exceeds $1,725,000. The practitioner who habitually uses this volume to look up the names of drugs with which to treat his patients is unwittingly being influenced in his therapeutic practice by nonmedical commercial interests. His very freedom of therapeutic practice is at risk. Yet many if not most doctors are unaware of this; here the leaders of the profession must be blamed because they have remained silent, an ironic omission for a leadership which has in recent times spent millions of dollars to fight forces they accuse of meddling in the "sacred doctor-patient relationship." It is my belief that there is no force in American life today which more directly meddles in this relationship than that segment of the pharmaceutical industry which operates through the detail man, through advertising, and most boldly of all, through the *Physicians' Desk Reference*.

Annual publication of *PDR* is an enterprise of Medical Economics, Inc., which distributes it without charge to over 200,000

[13] *Hearings on S. 1552*, Part 1, p. 137.

practicing "doctors of medicine and doctors of osteopathy." Until recently, it was also distributed free to "pharmacies and libraries of more than 5000 hospitals," but now these institutions have been asked to purchase their copies at a nominal cost. Doubtless most of them have done so, for of all the reference books located on hospital floors for the use of doctors and nurses, the one most often used by far is the *PDR*.

The *PDR* states that its contents have been obtained with the "cooperation" of drug manufacturers, through whose "patronage" its publication is made possible. This is euphemism. Drug houses *buy* space in the *PDR* and publish what they wish to publish. Even those unethical repackaging enterprises—"drug companies" owned and operated by physicians who buy up inexpensive generics, relabel them, and prescribe them under a special brand name at a higher price—are free to buy space. Since this is so, its contents can hardly be considered authoritative. *Precisely because it is an advertising catalogue, the PDR is incomplete; it gives prominent mention to too few generic names for widely consumed basic drugs.* The widespread use of this volume serves to conceal from practicing doctors the existence of numerous other manufacturers which very often can supply the same drugs at lower cost. There is a curious disclaimer in the foreword to *PDR* for 1960, the fourteenth annual edition: "It should be understood that in organizing the wealth of material in *PDR* the publisher is not advocating the use of any product listed by any manufacturer *nor attempting to influence the therapeutic practice of any physician.*" (My italics) In subsequent editions the italicized portion of the sentence was dropped.

The *Physicians' Desk Reference* has achieved its popularity not only by virtue of aggressive free distribution, but also because the profession itself offers no good alternative reference volume. I hope that the *Handbook* will meet the need for a brief authoritative list of essential basic prescription drugs which can be purchased at minimum cost.

The Reference Book Gap and the Role of the AMA

The *Handbook* would be incomplete without a mention of two authoritative volumes, *The Pharmacopeia of the United States of America* and *The National Formulary.* The former, usually designated as the *U.S.P.*, is published—at ten-year intervals since 1820 until very recently, when it began appearing at five-year intervals—by the private, scientific, nonprofit United States Pharmacopeial Convention, Inc., which exists for the sole purpose of providing up-to-date drug standards. The Convention is not dependent on drug company advertising and is in fact completely free of outside control or influence. Members of the board, officers, and those who serve on the Revision Committee have always been outstanding leaders in the fields of both pharmacy and medicine. With the passage in 1906 of the Pure Food and Drug Act, the *U.S.P.* was recognized by federal statute as an "official" compendium providing standards of strength, quality, and purity for the drugs it describes. Over the years the *U.S.P.* has listed only those drugs that reflect the best practice and teaching of medicine, decisions based on creditable and firmly grounded scientific fact. Thus, the *U.S.P.* is the single most valuable and reliable authority on the composition and quality of drugs. The most prestigious thing that can happen to a manufacturer's drug is its acceptance in the *U.S.P.*, where it is listed by its official, generic name.

It is most helpful for physicians to know which drugs are contained in the *U.S.P.* However, the volume is actually of limited value as a reference to the doctor at the moment when he prescribes medications, for it has not been designed to provide information on pharmacological activity, indications for use, manufacturers, and cost of the drugs.

Because the *U.S.P.* is subject to constant revision, drugs are always being demoted from it and others promoted to it. In consequence, some drugs may be excluded or dropped from the *U.S.P.* even though they are still widely used. In order to maintain a list of those drugs which are widely used but are not acceptable to the *U.S.P.*, the American Pharmaceutical Association publishes *The National Formulary*, often referred to simply as "the *N. F.*" The *N.F.*, whose format is similar to that of the *U.S.P.*, used to contain certain drugs simply because they were widely prescribed, but now it considers therapeutic worth and toxicity before inclusion. However, the *N.F.* will include mixtures of drugs, something which the *U.S.P.* will do only rarely since the prescription of mixtures and combinations of drugs is not generally considered the best therapeutic practice.

Because the doctor has never found it practical to use the *U.S.P.* and *N.F.* as reference books, the AMA used to publish an inexpensive and valuable volume known as the *Epitome of the U.S.P. and N.F.*, which listed the titles of the drugs in each volume and some useful facts about them. The discontinuation of this important service about fifteen years ago is partly responsible for the gap which the *PDR* has unfortunately filled.

Further responsibility for the gap lies with another decision of the AMA which discontinued publication in 1957 of an annual volume entitled *New and Nonofficial Remedies* (*N.N.R.*). The highly prestigious AMA Council on Pharmacy and Chemistry included in *N.N.R.* descriptions of many drugs not yet official either in the *N.F.* or the *U.S.P.* but deemed of sufficient importance and worth to describe to doctors. Conversely, the Council also included certain drugs which had achieved official status whenever it believed that the medical profession was not yet sufficiently well informed about them. Most reputable manufacturers used to apply to the justifiably influential Council to have their new products accepted. Drugs that were considered of little worth or those that carried a merchandising name or had been advertised in a misleading fashion were not likely to receive the approval of the Council, whose opinions were widely accepted and served a most valuable purpose. There is, incidentally, a "successor" to *New and Nonofficial Remedies* entitled *New Drugs*, an uncritical compilation of newly marketed agents which cannot be taken seriously as a guide to good prescribing practice.

The overwhelming number of practicing doctors are single-mindedly concerned with giving their patients the most effective medication with the least possible chance of unwanted side effect or toxicity. Most doctors—like most people of any kind—are likely to be suspicious that a bargain may be cut-rate in quality as well as cost. There may even be a matching tendency to believe that something more expensive must also be of higher quality.

While honest skepticism is always healthy, such attitudes may be misleading. A quotation from the *Nebraska State Medical Journal*, cited in *Drug News Weekly* of January 31, 1966, asks: "Is it through no accident that cheap has come to mean inferior as well as inexpensive?" The question was asked in the context of a discussion as to the advisability of prescribing by generic name. This seemingly sensible attitude is buttressed by editorial comment in the *Journal of the American Medical Association:*[14] ". . . the physician who prescribes meprobamate[15] as such has no way of knowing that his patient will receive the drug in a form of highest quality and expected potency." The AMA did

[14] Editorial, "Drug Names," Vol. CXC, No. 6 (November 9, 1964), p. 542.

[15] Meprobamate is the generic name for a widely advertised sedative most commonly bought as Miltown® and Equanil®.

not always take this stand, however; until only recently, the AMA was on record as favoring the use of generic names in preference to brand names.[16] The preference for generic names was based on the belief that "this would avoid much needless tax on memory with its attendant confusion and errors." Dr. Austin Smith, when he was secretary of the Council on Pharmacy and Chemistry of the AMA in 1944, wrote: "One of the greatest evils of the use of protected names [i.e., brand names, which are trademarked] lies in the confusion they create. The old story of methenamine being prescribed in one prescription under six different names is a standing joke in materia medica classes, and yet other examples just as questionable are evident in everyday practice." Elsewhere in the same article Dr. Smith told of "a large hospital in an eastern city [which] did away with the expense of prescribing proprietary agents when official counterparts were available, and unnecessarily complex mixtures and the absurd practice of prescribing names instead of therapeutically active agents. This pharmacy within one year effected a saving of $50,000."[17]

To avoid the proliferation of brand names, the *Journal of the American Medical Association* used to permit only the originator of a product to advertise under a brand name in AMA periodicals, while all other purveyors were required to use the generic name instead of their own brand names. Quoting the late Senator Kefauver: "The effect of these requirements was generally to curtail advertising excesses in the prescription field. Doctors relied heavily on the AMA *Journal* to keep abreast of new drug products, and most manufacturers found it worth while to place their advertising where it counted. The Council's [Council on

[16] American Medical Association, *New and Nonofficial Remedies 1950*, Official Rules of the Council, Rule 4, p. xix.

[17] Austin Smith, "The Council on Pharmacy and Chemistry," *The Journal of the American Medical Association*, Vol. CXXIV, No. 7 (February 12, 1944), p. 435.

Pharmacy and Chemistry of the AMA] controls also tended to maintain some competitive balance between the large and small units in the industry. The Seal of Acceptance [indicating approval by the Council] was very important to small manufacturers; it was prominently displayed as proof positive to physicians that the product was of high quality. The fact that only the originator of a new product could use a brand name was also a marked asset; for the small company there was a decided prestige element in the recognition that it was the contributor of the development."[18]

Sadly, the AMA attitude changed shortly thereafter; its policies were reversed in the mid-1950s after it hired the Chicago firm of Ben Gaffin & Associates, Inc., to research ways of improving the sale of advertising space in the *JAMA*. Whether related or not, it is a fact that the fifty-eight-year-old Council Seal of Acceptance Program was shelved, publication of a small volume called *Useful Drugs*, whose wide use had the effect of "ensuring both safe and effective use of drugs as well as limiting their number through authoritative suggestion,"[19] was discontinued, and consideration of advertising was taken out of the jurisdiction of the eminent Council on Pharmacy and Chemistry and placed in the hands of an advertising committee. AMA advertising revenues suddenly increased dramatically, but in the words of one distinguished professor of medicine, "they lost the most valuable tool they ever had as far as being of service to the profession, and clearly appreciated by the public."[20] Thus it was that the Council on Pharmacy and Chemistry lost its position of authority, contributing to the vacuum which has ever since been filled by the pharmaceutical manufacturers.

[18] Estes Kefauver, *In a Few Hands* (New York, Pantheon Books, 1965), p. 74.

[19] Dr. Walter Modell, Editorial, *Clinical Pharmacology and Therapeutics*, Vol. II, No. 1 (January–February 1961).

[20] Kefauver, *In a Few Hands*, pp. 76–77.

The Move to Promote Generic Prescribing, and the Reaction

Many responsible members of our government are aware of the large savings to be made by buying generic rather than brand-name drugs where possible, and plans are under way to introduce legislation requiring the dispensing of generic preparations to patients whose drugs are being paid for under tax-supported Medicare. This comes as no surprise to those who know that all the military medical facilities buy and dispense only drugs which are bought by the Defense Supply Agency of the United States government under generic names from the lowest competitive bidders (Appendix A). Although many of the contract winners are small and middle-sized manufacturers (*institutional* buyers such as municipal hospitals are at present their major market), when the big corporations have entered into sealed bidding there have been some remarkable revelations. For example, CIBA, the enormous Switzerland-based company, offered to sell to the United States government for about 60 cents a quantity and quality of reserpine (1000 0.25 mgm tablets) for which the corner pharmacist must pay $39.50. The government buys it as (generic name) "reserpine"; the corner pharmacist buys and dispenses it as (brand name) "Serpasil." There are no important differences between the two; only the name—and $39. Ironically, CIBA did not win the contract, for they were underbid by a company willing to sell the same drug for 51 cents.

In addition to federal government institutions, state and municipal and many private nonprofit hospitals buy generics. Many have their own formulary, which restricts in-hospital usage to a list of selected basic generic drugs, the appropriate one being substituted for the expensive brand-name item wherever the institution's own committee on drugs (consisting of its own physicians and pharmacists) deems it appropriate and suitable. This meets with nearly unanimous acceptance on the part of the doctors, but is anathema to brand-name manufacturers. According to corporate thinking, the formulary restricts the doctor's freedom of choice. Therefore the National Pharmaceutical Council, Inc. (NPC), whose relatively few dues-paying members are exclusively heavily advertised brand-name drug manufacturers, is, according to its executive vice president (who appeared before the Kefauver Subcommittee in May 1960), "particularly concerned with the practice known as substitution." He went on to say: ". . . a physician, in prescribing a particular brand of drug for a patient, may be doing so because that brand has characteristics which the physician wants his patient to have and which may not be present in other brands. The generic name does not indicate to the dispensing pharmacist what these characteristics are and he cannot necessarily tell from reading the prescription why the prescriber chose the brand he did. If the pharmacist is permitted to substitute the so-called generic equivalent, he *very likely* is not substituting a drug with equivalent characteristics and may be defeating the very purpose of the physician in selecting the brand of drug he chose."[21]

The statement is nonsense. In seventeen years of clinical experience, an instance where a prescription was written for a brand-name drug because of "characteristics" other than the identity of its major ingredient has never come to my attention. Furthermore, close physician colleagues I have questioned are unaware of any such instances. The representative of the National Pharmaceutical Council ended his prepared remarks by asserting: ". . . we insist that the medical profession be left free to prescribe exactly what it sees fit and that the public be assured that it gets what the doctor prescribed."[22] Any implication that the generically named drug does not contain what the doctor prescribed is false.

The Council proposed to spend $140,498 in 1960 alone to

[21] *Hearings on S. Res. 238*, Part 21, pp. 11695, 11699.
[22] *Ibid.*, p. 11701.

protect this "freedom" of doctors. It is difficult not to believe that the National Pharmaceutical Council is in reality prepared to spend large sums of money to perpetuate and exploit a situation which many in the medical profession (and a growing number of lay persons) find distasteful, viz. the undue influence which multimillion-dollar promotion has applied to the practicing doctor and to the public. With the assistance and prodding of the National Pharmaceutical Council, the majority of the fifty individual state pharmacy boards have influenced state legislatures to adopt resolutions prohibiting a pharmacist from substituting one brand-name drug or a generic-name drug for another. This has taken place quietly; doubtless few citizens are aware of it. Of course, the Council is not entirely successful: the Director of Drugs and Drug Stores of Michigan, Mr. O. K. Grettenberger, testified before the Kefauver Subcommittee that an attempt by the Michigan State Board of Pharmacy to suspend the license of a pharmacist, one E. L. Casden, for filling a prescription for Meticorten with another brand of prednisone instead was not justified under law. A state court found that "chemically and by assay the drugs were identical."[23] Meticorten is the Schering Corporation's form of prednisone, and is often ten times as costly as prednisone sold by generic name or even by other brand names.[24]

The druggist, himself the object of advertisements and of the "educating" salesmen, in his honest desire to be a helpful, reliable partner of the doctor passes along to him dark rumors of generically named drug tablets which do not dissolve in the gastrointestinal tract (a phenomenon which must be very difficult to document) and remarkable testimonial anecdotes of his own as to the impotence of generic penicillin (classically about a patient with fever, treated with generic penicillin G without apparent effect, who improves only after the doctor switches

[23] *Hearings on S. Res. 238*, Part 21, pp. 11592–93.
[24] *Ibid.*

to a brand-name penicillin G). Doctors are human, and while they may recognize that such stories are usually impossible to prove and often lacking in logic, the seeds of doubt may be planted and take root—for after all, is it not axiomatic that quality always costs a little more? Did not the National Pharmaceutical Council distribute a pamphlet listing twenty-four "reasons" why brand names should be specified on prescription blanks? This pamphlet was even made available as a handout in drugstores; unfortunately, a brilliant point-by-point dissection of this fatuous document, made before Senate Subcommittee hearings by Dr. Walter Modell, the distinguished Professor of Therapeutics at Cornell Medical School and the New York Hospital, goes unread.[25] The campaign to make doctors and patients ill at ease about prescribing and using generic drugs has been highly successful; prejudice against the use of generics is deeply instilled and will be overcome only gradually.

The big brand-name drug houses, through their executives and representatives, openly disparage products sold as generics and undoubtedly influence some doctors to adopt a similar view. For example, I received a "Dear Doctor" letter from the vice president in charge of sales of one of the largest corporations; the letter began: "Although there is nothing unusual about substandard drugs being sold by small manufacturers lacking quality-control procedures . . ."

The entire incident surrounding this letter deserves extended comment, for it is rich in revelation. The letter was in response to my request for further information regarding the allegation made by his detail man that a United States government agency had unwittingly bought substandard digoxin. While disowning knowledge of the allegation, the vice president did make reference to three recorded instances in which substandard digoxin was, in fact, sold by two small companies. He enclosed a reproduction of an article from *The Brooklyn Eagle* of January 1963

[25] *Hearings on S. Res. 238*, Part 21, pp. 11608–27.

describing a "Crack-Down on Heart Drug as Too Weak" and "seizure" of digoxin tablets from two Manhattan drugstores, and also enclosed a pamphlet published by the National Pharmaceutical Council. In the first place, the disparaging reference to generic manufacturers was uncalled for, since there is reason to believe, as will be shown later, that the word "big" could have been used as meaningfully as "small" in describing manufacturers who produce substandard products. Second, since digoxin is sold generically by more than fifty small companies, it makes no more sense to blackball all of them for the quality-control slips of two than it would be to blackball the vice president's corporation for the recorded quality-control slips of other brand-name manufacturers. The presentation of material of this nature to a physician searching for a factual report shows surprising evasion and irresponsibility.

Finally, the NPC pamphlet "Misconceptions about So-called 'Generic Equivalent' Drugs" is worth analysis. Its general thesis is that there is no such thing as a "generic equivalent" because in addition to the major ingredient in a tablet or capsule, there are also inert substances: bases to create bulk, absorbents, disintegrants, and binders to hold the tablet together. The pamphlet implies that the know-how required to produce a tablet or capsule which will disintegrate properly and release the active drug is somehow unlikely to be the possession of those who manufacture generic drugs. To be sure, there are incompetent manufacturers who have marketed improperly compounded tablets which do not, for example, disintegrate as they should, but the information supplied in the *Handbook* will make it possible for doctor, patient, and pharmacist to buy generic drugs with a high degree of assurance that they meet the specifications of the *United States Pharmacopeia.* As a matter of fact, all important techniques of drug compounding are common knowledge and within the ability of any conscientious manufacturer, large or small. Most of these techniques are among the oldest arts of medicine. The substances used as bases are milk sugar, salt, starch, and a simple sugar, mannitol. For absorbents both milk sugar and starch will do. As a disintegrator, cornstarch is the popular choice and works well. Binders in general use are gelatine, gum acacia, gum tragacanth, molasses, dextrin, and less commonly, cellulose. Physicians and lay persons alike will recognize all of these substances as inert materials about which there can be little mystery. As for modern tablet-making machines, they are available to anyone wishing to buy them. (The interested reader can find excellent brief monographs on tablet making and tablet coating in any pharmacy library.)

The NPC pamphlet is correct in stating that there is no generic name for tablets or capsules which contain two or more active drugs. However, this is because the *United States Pharmacopeia* does not include combinations and nearly every teacher of pharmacology and clinical medicine discourages their use, and with good reason. A tablet or capsule containing a mixture of drugs limits the doctor to a fixed dosage ratio. Nevertheless, in support of such combinations the pamphlet states categorically that it is "more economical to prescribe a single preparation than to prescribe separate ingredients by generic names." This does not agree with my observations. (See "Drugs for High Blood Pressure" and "Drugs for Gastrointestinal Disorders.")

The Council pamphlet refers in passing to the "minimum requirements" of the *United States Pharmacopeia*, subtly implying that *U.S.P.* standards can be exceeded or bettered, and some readers could infer from it that brand-name drugs do just that and generics do not. For example, with respect to the matter of dosage, it happens that the human body is not delicately sensitive to small variations in dosage of most drugs.[26] Therefore, in many cases the *U.S.P.* permits the weight of a tablet to vary some-

[26] An illustration of this fortunate degree of tolerance is in the almost universal practice of giving adults the same dose of most drugs without respect to body weight.

what. Thus, a tablet stated to contain 100 milligrams of a drug may in some cases contain as little as 95 or as much as 105 milligrams. Exceeding 105 milligrams can be as potentially serious as failing to provide 95 milligrams. It makes no sense to think in terms of "exceeding" the dosage requirements of the *U.S.P.*

"Why do so many physicians specify drugs by brands?" asks the Council, which proceeds to answer its own query in part by saying of generic drugs: "The patient taking such a drug may suffer an unexpected reaction, not experienced with the drug with which the physician is familiar containing the same active agent. Is the reaction due to the drug or to some inert ingredient used by the maker as a flavoring agent, binder, or for other purposes of dosage formulation?" Now, allergic reactions can *theoretically* occur from these substances (although I have never personally seen one), but there is no basis for believing that a flavoring agent, base, absorbent, disintegrant, or binder used by a manufacturer of generic drugs is any more likely to cause allergy than one used by a manufacturer of brand-name drugs. Actually, allergy to a medication is nearly always due to its *major* ingredient and for this reason a strong argument can be made for referring to drugs by generic name. In many cases the same drug has several very different-sounding brand names:[27] if a patient had shown an allergy to this drug under one brand name and the physician switched him to another brand without realizing that it was the same drug, the result would be continuation or worsening of the allergic reaction.

Having nearly rested its case, the National Pharmaceutical Council pamphlet takes up the matter of prescriptions written for welfare patients: "Some individuals take the position that prescriptions for welfare patients should be written generically, on the theory that some public funds presumably will be conserved, and that 'generic equivalent' drugs are good enough for

[27] Syncillin, Darcil, Alpen, Chemipen, Dramcillin, and Maxipen are all brand names for a particular kind of penicillin.

the patient who cannot pay for them. Are reasons which dictate a physician's choice of a reliable brand-name drug for a sick patient any less valid because the patient cannot pay for the best treatment available? Are there in fact tremendous savings to be achieved by relegating the welfare patient to the class of second-rate citizen?" The Council has an admirably sensitive social conscience, but it is reminded that when the President of the United States, a senator, a representative, or any other high government official becomes ill and is hospitalized at Walter Reed Hospital or the United States Naval Hospital in Bethesda, Maryland, he is treated with drugs bought by generic name from approximately one hundred different companies of which only about twenty are large and well-known manufacturers.[28] Is there any reason why other citizens should not have access to these same medications?

What About Research?

There is merit to the argument that some large pharmaceutical companies do important research and maintain facilities to provide a number of public services for which they are never adequately compensated in dollars. On the other hand, few manufacturers of generic drugs do research and none is equipped to provide an adequate supply, let us say, of rare antitoxins should need ever arise, whereas some of the big companies are in a position to do so. It has been pointed out, however, that the large corporations spend nearly four times as much for advertising and promotion as they do for research, and it has been said that much of the latter takes the form of "molecule-manipulating" attempts to produce a drug which will have the same pharmacological effect as an agent already patented and marketed by a competitor. Upon discovering such a compound the company

[28] Senate Report No. 448, p. 247.

may patent it, market it, and join in the competition even though the new drug offers no substantial advantage over the older, better-known one. (The reader is referred to the Prescription Drug List, Section XI, pages 127–32, which deals with many similar oral diuretics.) It is the proliferation of such drugs, each with its own brand name, each launched with a giant promotional campaign, that has caused much of the confusion besetting the doctor. Activity of this sort could conceivably be beneficial by giving rise to price competition. Unfortunately, this rarely happens because the major manufacturers, with a few exceptions, peg their prices at practically the same, often identical figures.

However, while one can therefore legitimately question the value of introducing "copy-cat" drugs, it is not entirely fair to question the kind of research (viz., molecule manipulating) which makes them available. Anyone aware of the nature of pharmacology knows it is impossible to predict when a small change in molecular structure is going to cause significant beneficial change in pharmacological effect or in toxicity. (A mere increase in potency is not beneficial, however, for it makes little difference to the patient whether he swallows a 10 or a 500 milligram tablet.) There is no doubt that the pharmaceutical industry has made many important research contributions.[29] Many conscientious physicians undoubtedly feel that this one factor alone justifies prescribing brand-name items even though the patents have expired and patients have to pay more than if generic equivalents are prescribed. There is something to be said for this view, *provided public money is not involved* (*as with welfare or Medicare patients*) *and that private patients who foot drug bills directly are agreeable. Patients* (*who are "captive consumers"*) *have a right to know for what services they are paying.* Other equally conscientious physicians may take the view that

[29] About two thirds of the *Handbook's* basic drugs were developed entirely or in part by the pharmaceutical industry, but the patents by now have expired on more than half of these.

the responsibility of the doctor is to his patient's immediate welfare—including his pocketbook—and may not wish to allow an ideology of sorts to influence therapeutic practice.

The Substantive and Crucial Question: Are Brand-Name Products Superior?

It is the contention of the *Handbook* that no one is in a position to make ironclad guarantees for any manufactured product, drugs included, and that there is no good reason to believe that brand-name drugs are necessarily more reliable than generics as to quality, purity, and potency. There is compelling evidence for this view in Table 1 (pages 36–71), which presents unabridged details of all drug recalls[30] during a thirty-three month period ending June 30, 1965. This information was supplied by the Food and Drug Administration to a congressional committee. The facts speak for themselves: *nearly half of the recalls involved products of the largest and best-known corporations.* It is plain that a pharmaceutical manufacturer's reliability is not related either to size or to advertising budget. One wonders even whether physician, pharmacist, and patient have not been placing exaggerated confidence in certain well-known firms. It would be incorrect to infer that all large pharmaceutical manufacturers are not reliable in their over-all production, but the evidence does point up the injustice in wholesale condemnation of all smaller drug manufacturers.

Because 90 percent of the drugs currently sold in the United States are produced by about two dozen of the largest brand-name drug manufacturers, it is fair to ask whether the number of their substandard products, accounting for nearly half of the total in Table 1, is nonetheless disproportionately smaller than

[30] The removal from a pharmacy of drugs discovered not to meet *U.S.P.* standards or of drugs which are mislabeled.

would be expected. It is possible to provide a tentative answer, since the Kefauver Subcommittee did its work so thoroughly. In the hearings the then Commissioner of Food and Drugs, Mr. George Larrick, testified: "We confine sampling to drugs which we have reason to believe may be misbranded or adulterated."[31] Mr. Larrick provided data showing the number of samples taken per one-million-dollar volume of business in the cases of several large and several small companies during the decade 1950–1960. In the cases of Merck, CIBA, Schering, and Carter Products (Wallace Laboratories), one sample alone was taken per one million dollars of business; for Smith Kline & French, Lederle, Pfizer, and Upjohn the range was from one to less than five per one million dollars. For small companies, however, the situation was strikingly different, for here the number of samples ranged around one hundred per one million dollars and in several instances was even more numerous![32] This kind of sampling, in effect, spotlights the violations of the small companies, upon which the enforcement work is concentrated.

Furthermore, with respect to the activities of the major drug companies, Dr. Barbara Moulton, formerly an FDA staff member, testified: "Private conferences between representatives of industry and the Food and Drug Administration staff members are also the rule rather than the exception with respect to regulatory action under the law." Thus, when a large manufacturer was concerned, situations more commonly than not were rectified by informal rather than official agreement. Thus, damaging reports of official recall actions were often avoided, for the FDA records of such informal agreements were allegedly incomplete.[33]

Not least of the reasons forcing us to believe that brand-name drugs are not necessarily better than those sold by generic names is a finding made in the spring of 1966 by the United States Food

[31] *Hearings on S. 1552*, Part 22, p. 12113.
[32] Senate Report No. 448, p. 246.
[33] *Ibid.*

and Drug Administration. At the direction of its new, no-nonsense Commissioner, Dr. James Goddard, the Agency sampled 4600 drugs from 250 manufacturers. Quoting Mr. Winton B. Rankin, Deputy Commissioner, as he addressed the American College of Apothecaries on October 15, 1966, in Boston, Massachusetts: "About 2600 of the drugs were sold by their generic name only and about 2000 by brand name. They represented 20 of the most important groups of drugs used in medicine—antihypertensives, oral antidiabetics, anti-infectives, digitalis and digitalis-like preparations, for example. Antibiotics were not included because every lot of antibiotics for human use is checked by FDA before sale." Deputy Commissioner Rankin then went on to reveal to a hushed audience of pharmacists that "7.8 percent of the generic-named drugs were not of acceptable potency, 8.8 percent of the brand-named drugs were not of acceptable potency." Later, in reply to a question from the audience, the speaker made it clear that the difference between the 7.8 and 8.8 percent figures is not large enough to allow one to conclude that generic drugs are necessarily better than those sold by brand name.

Table 1: *Lists of Drug Recalls and Other Actions Under the Good Manufacturing Practices Section of the Food, Drug, and Cosmetic Act*

List I

Drug Recalls (Requested or Voluntary), January 1 to June 30, 1965

FIRM	PRODUCT	DATE	REASON
Philips Roxane, Inc., St. Louis, Mo.	Aero Mast	1/5/65	Low potency
G & W Labs, Inc., Jersey City, N.J.	Aminophylline 7½ gr suppositories	1/12/65	1 pkg of 1002 sup. labeled Aspirin 10 gr
McKesson & Robbins, Bridgeport, Conn.	Tetracycline Syrup 125 mg/5 cc	1/12/65	Gas formation in product
Nysco Labs, Inc., Long Island City, N.Y.	Pot. Penicillin G Tabs 100,000 units	1/19/65	Low potency
Zenith Labs, Inc., Englewood, N.J.	Penicillin Tabs 400,000 units	1/25/65	High moisture
Maizel Labs, Inc., Chicago, Ill.	Atropine Injection	1/15/65	Label mixup
Medical Chemical Corp., Chicago, Ill.	Atropate Injection (pentobarbital inj.)	1/19/65	Label mixup
Rachel Laboratories, Long Beach, Calif.	Tetracycline Syrup	1/26/65	Gas formation in syrup
S. E. Massengill Co., Bristol, Tenn.	Bethramin Elixir 15%	1/26/65	Low potency of B_{12}

Disposition of Cases Code

[1] Citations (only eight citation decisions made to date in List II). The cases marked are the only ones in which there were citations.

[2] Prosecution recommended to General Counsel

[3] Prosecution pending

[4] Prosecuted

[5] Pending

[6] Temporary Abeyance

[7] Permanent Abeyance

FIRM	PRODUCT	DATE	REASON
Atlas Pharm. Labs, Inc., Detroit, Mich.	Progesterone Suspension 25 mg/cc 10 cc vials	1/27/65	Nonsterile
Diamond Labs, Inc., Des Moines, Iowa	Cortasep #1	1/27/65	Label mixup
Maurry Biological Co., Los Angeles, Calif.	Prednisolone 25 mg	1/27/65	Label mixup
Maizel Labs, Inc., Chicago, Ill.	Pentobarbital Injection 2 gr	1/20/65	Label mixup
Maizel Labs, Inc., Chicago, Ill.	Pentobarbital Sodium Injection 2 gr	2/2/65	Label mixup
Merck Sharp & Dohme, West Point, Pa.	Alflorone Topical Lotion 0.1%	2/1/65	Low potency
K-V Pharmacal Co., St. Louis, Mo.	Apap Tabs (acetaminophen)	2/1/65	Low potency
Upjohn Company, Kalamazoo, Mich.	Propylthiouracil Tabs	2/4/65	Penicillin contamination
Upjohn Company, Kalamazoo, Mich.	PAC Caps	2/4/65	Penicillin contamination
Armour Laboratories, Kankakee, Ill.	Alpha Chymar 750 unit/vials	2/4/65	Excess moisture Low potency
Pilco Laboratories, Cedar Rapids, Iowa	Thyroid 1 gr tabs	2/8/65	Label mixup
Standard Pharmacal Co., Elgin, Ill.	Pulvex Tapeworm Tabs	2/8/65	Label mixup Printing error
Upjohn Company, Kalamazoo, Mich.	Neomycin Nyastatin Tabs	2/8/65	Low potency
Upjohn Company, Detroit, Mich.	Digitora 1.28 gr	2/9/65	Penicillin contamination
Merck Sharpe & Dohme, West Point, Pa.	Hydropres 25 mg	2/10/65	Label mixup

FIRM	PRODUCT	DATE	REASON
Eli Lilly & Co., Indianapolis, Ind.	Streptomycin Sulfate Prod. 431 & 692	2/12/65	Penicillin contamination
Eli Lilly & Co., Indianapolis, Ind.	Ilotycin Glucoheptonate I.V. 500 mg & 1 gm ampules	2/12/65	Penicillin contamination
C. M. Bundy Co., Cincinnati, Ohio	Hydrocort	2/5/65	Label mixup
Masti-Kure Products Co., Norwich, Conn.	Masti-Kure	2/5/65	Low potency
Zenith Labs, Inc., Englewood, N.J.	Royal Jelly 50 mg caps	2/17/65	Penicillin contamination
Zenith Labs, Inc., Englewood, N.J.	APC Tabs, green #2	2/17/65	Penicillin contamination
Zenith Labs, Inc., Englewood, N.J.	Aspirin 5 gr tabs	2/17/65	Penicillin contamination
Generic Drugs, Pennsauken, N.J.	Bevite 1000 (B_{12} inj.) 10 cc vials	3/3/65	Label mix-up. mg instead of mcg
Chas. Pfizer & Co., New York, N.Y.	Terramycin I.M. 10 cc	3/4/65	Label mix-up. Vial carton mislabeled "Strep-Combiotic"
Morton Pharmaceuticals, Inc.,[1,7] Memphis, Tenn.	Salicylamide Tabs 4 gr	3/5/65	Low potency
Lakeside Labs, Inc., Milwaukee, Wis.	Glaucon (sol. levo-epinephrine)	3/10/65	Black particles in sterile solution
Philadelphia Labs, Philadelphia, Pa.	Bacitracin 50,000 units/ml	3/15/65	Low potency

FIRM	PRODUCT	DATE	REASON
Schering Corporation, Bloomfield, N.J.	Fulvicin (griseofulvin) Tabs 500 mg	3/15/65	Penicillin contamination
Ankh Labs, Inc., Fairborn, Ohio	Ankh Plate Tops	3/16/65	Low potency
Abbott Laboratories, N. Chicago, Ill.	Erythrocin Sulfa Chewable Tabs	3/16/65	Penicillin contamination
Abbott Laboratories, N. Chicago, Ill.	Pediamycin Sulfa Chewable Tabs	3/16/65	Penicillin contamination
Parke, Davis & Co., Detroit, Mich.	Humatin Paromomycin	3/18/65	Penicillin contamination
Chas. Pfizer & Co., New York, N.Y.	Cortril Acetate Aqueous Suspension 5 cc (hydrocortisone)	3/22/65	Particles adhering to side
Philadelphia Labs, Philadelphia, Pa.	Triple Sulfa Tabs	3/16/65	Penicillin contamination
Davis-Edwards Pharmacal Co., New York, N.Y.	Prednisolone Tabs	3/31/65	Low potency
Lakeside Labs, Inc., Milwaukee, Wis.	Caytine Aerosol Inhalers with phenylephrine	3/31/65	Wrong ingredient
Lit Drug Company,[1,7] Newark, N.J.	Aspirin 5 gr tabs	4/5/65	Decomposed
Zenith Labs, Inc., Englewood, N.J.	Meprobamate 400 mg tabs	4/5/65	Penicillin contamination
Ciba Pharmaceutical Co., Summit, N.J.	Vinactane (viomycin SO_4) Injection	4/6/65	Penicillin contamination
Johnson & Johnson, Chicago, Ill.	Absorbent Dental Points	4/6/65	Nonsterile

FIRM	PRODUCT	DATE	REASON
Integrity Magnesia Corp., Philadelphia, Pa.	Blue Seal Citrate of Magnesia	4/6/65	Label mix-up. Contains rubbing alcohol
Philips Roxane, Inc., St. Joseph, Mo.	Mepine Injection 10 cc vials	4/6/65	Low potency
Pure Labs, Inc. Parsippany, N.J.	Streptomycin SO_4 1 gm & 5 gm vials	4/7/65	Penicillin contamination
Supreme Pharmaceutical Co., Inc., Jersey City, N.J.	Methyl Testosterone sublingual tab 10 mg	4/7/65	Penicillin contamination
Strong Cobb Arner, Inc., Cleveland, Ohio	Phenobarbital ¼ gr tab	4/9/65	Penicillin contamination
Merck Sharp & Dohme, West Point, Pa.	Cortisone Acetate Ophthalmic Sol. 2.5%	4/9/65	Label mix-up. Outer cartons labeled Hydrocortisone Sol. 0.5%
Philadelphia Labs, Philadelphia, Pa.	Antacid Tabs	4/9/65	Penicillin contamination
Philadelphia Labs, Philadelphia, Pa.	Kolital Tabs	4/9/65	Penicillin contamination
McKesson & Robbins, Bridgeport, Conn.	Meprobamate	4/12/65	Penicillin contamination
McKesson & Robbins, Bridgeport, Conn.	Prednisolone	4/12/65	Penicillin contamination
Wm. S. Merrell Co., Cincinnati, Ohio	Benolone (15 mg/-15 ml bentyl)	4/13/65	Variation in potency
Eli Lilly & Co., Indianapolis, Ind.	H. T. Morphine Sulfate ⅛ gr & ⅙ gr	4/15/65	Label mixup

FIRM	PRODUCT	DATE	REASON
Chas. Pfizer & Co., New York, N.Y.	Viocin 1 gm vials	4/16/65	Penicillin contamination
Chas. Pfizer & Co., New York, N.Y.	Terramycin Intravenous 500 mg vials	4/16/65	Penicillin contamination
Chas. Pfizer & Co., New York, N.Y.	Tetracyn Intravenous 250 mg vials	4/16/65	Penicillin contamination
Chas. Pfizer & Co., New York, N.Y.	Tetracyn Intravenous 500 mg vials	4/16/65	Penicillin contamination
Chas. Pfizer & Co., New York, N.Y.	Tetracyn Intramuscular 250 mg vials	4/16/65	Penicillin contamination
Chas. Pfizer & Co., New York, N.Y.	Tetracyn Intramuscular 100 mg vials	4/16/65	Penicillin contamination
Chas. Pfizer & Co., New York, N.Y.	Terracydin Caps	4/16/65	Penicillin contamination
Chas. Pfizer & Co., New York, N.Y.	Niamid Tabs 100 mg.	4/16/65	Penicillin contamination
Chas. Pfizer & Co., New York, N.Y.	Niamid Tabs 25 mg	4/16/65	Penicillin contamination
Chas. Pfizer & Co., New York, N.Y.	Moderil Tabs 0.25 mg	4/16/65	Penicillin contamination
Chas. Pfizer & Co., New York, N.Y.	Neobiotic Tabs 500 mg	4/16/65	Penicillin contamination
Chas. Pfizer & Co., New York, N.Y.	Polymyxin B Sulfate Sterile Powder 50 mg vials	4/16/65	Penicillin contamination

/ Table 1: Lists of Drug Recalls

FIRM	PRODUCT	DATE	REASON
Chas. Pfizer & Co., New York, N.Y.	Oleandomycin Intramuscular 200 mg vials	4/16/65	Penicillin contamination
Chas. Pfizer & Co., New York, N.Y.	Oleandomycin Parenteral 500 mg vials	4/16/65	Penicillin contamination
Chas. Pfizer & Co., New York, N.Y.	Tao Caps 250 mg	4/16/65	Penicillin contamination
Chas. Pfizer & Co., New York, N.Y.	Streptomycin Sulfate 1 & 5 gm vials	4/16/65	Penicillin contamination
Physicians Products Co., Petersburg, Va.	Transerpine 0.25 mg	4/28/65	Penicillin contamination
Philadelphia Labs, Philadelphia, Pa.	Sulfadiazine Tabs 7.7 gr	4/28/65	Penicillin contamination
Sherman Laboratories, Detroit, Mich.	Urakon Dextrose Solution	4/23/65	Variation in potency
Lit Drug Company,[1,7] Newark, N.J.	Reserpine .5 mg tabs	4/29/65	Foreign alkaloids
Lit Drug Company,[1,7] Newark, N.J.	Sodium Salicylate 5 gr	4/29/65	Fails disintegration tests
Lit Drug Company,[1,7] Newark, N.J.	Ferrous Sulfate 5 gr	4/29/65	Low potency
Lit Drug Company,[1,7] Newark, N.J.	Triple Sulfa Tabs	4/29/65	Low potency
Lit Drug Company,[1,7] Newark, N.J.	Sulfadiazine Tabs 5 gr	4/29/65	Fails disintegration tests
Proctor & Gamble Co., Dayton, Ohio	Head & Shoulders Shampoo	4/30/65	Contaminated with pseudomonas

FIRM	PRODUCT	DATE	REASON
Rabin-Winters Corp., El Segundo, Calif.	F-M Vitamins, therapeutic geriatric	5/3/65	Improper label. Did not contain menadione
Jensen Salsbery Labs, Kansas City, Mo.	Pen FZ (proc. pen. G with nitrofurazone)	5/5/65	Low potency
Reid Provident Lab., Hialeah, Fla.	Tokisan Spray	5/12/65	Low potency
Bristol-Myers Co., Hillside, N.J.	Excedrin	5/13/65	Label mixup
Wyeth Laboratories, Evanston, Ill.	Oxaine-M	5/26/65	Clumps & discoloration

Drug Recalls (Requested or Voluntary), January 1 to December 31, 1964

FIRM	PRODUCT	DATE	REASON
E. R. Squibb & Sons,[1,7] Brooklyn, N.Y.	Aspirin 5000 tab bottles	1/7/64	Product mixup. Some bottles contain penicillin tabs
E. R. Squibb & Sons,[1,7] Brooklyn, N.Y.	Theragran Multi-Vitamin	1/10/64	Ingredient substitution. Niacin substituted for niacinamide
E. R. Squibb & Sons, Brooklyn, N.Y.	Rutorbin 50's Kenacort 100's	1/15/64	Packaging mixup. One bottle Rutorbin (correctly labeled) found in carton labeled Kenacort

FIRM	PRODUCT	DATE	REASON
Hoffmann-LaRoche, Inc., Nutley, N.J.	Madribon (Sulfa) 0.5 gm tablets	1/15/64	Label mix-up. Some bottles labeled Madribon Chewable 0.25 gm
Richlyn Labs, Inc., Philadelphia, Pa.	Heparin Sodium 1000 u/cc	1/23/64	Excess potency
Richlyn Labs, Inc., Philadelphia, Pa.	Digoxin 0.25 mg tabs	1/27/64	Wide variation in potency of individual tabs
Case Laboratories, Chicago, Ill.	Nystatin Sensitivity Discs	2/13/64	Low potency
Dixie Laboratories,[1,7] Seagoville, Texas	Mineral Oil 16 oz–32 oz	2/15/64	Contaminated with isopropyl alcohol
E. R. Squibb & Sons, Brooklyn, N.Y.	Mystecline F Caps	2/25/64	Low potency
E. R. Squibb & Sons,[1,7] Brooklyn, N.Y.	Theragran-M (vitamin-mineral)	2/25/64	Ingredient substitution. Niacin substituted for niacinamide
E. R. Squibb & Sons,[1,7] Brooklyn, N.Y.	Vesprin (triflupromazine)	2/25/64	Low potency
E. R. Squibb & Sons, Brooklyn, N.Y.	Stilbetin 0.10 mg tabs	2/25/64	Low potency
Richlyn Labs, Inc., Philadelphia, Pa.	Digoxin 0.25 mg tabs	3/9/64	Substantial variation in individual tablet potency

FIRM	PRODUCT	DATE	REASON
Merck & Co., Inc., Rahway, N.J.	Sodium Phosphate NF 1 lb	3/13/64	Label mix-up. Sodium phosphate labeled as Potassium Chloride
Merck Sharp & Dohme, West Point, Pa.	Aramine and Alpharedisol	1/27/64	Label mix-up. Some cartons Aramine labeled as Alpharedisol
E. R. Squibb & Sons, Brooklyn, N.Y.	Kenalog Orabase 5 gm tubes	3/16/64	Label mix-up. Some tubes labeled Kenalog Ointment
E. R. Squibb & Sons, Brooklyn, N.Y.	Phenobarbital ½ gr tabs	3/16/64	Excess potency
Durel Pharmaceutical Co., Mount Vernon, N.Y.	Durel-Cort Lotion-Ointment	4/2/64	Variation in potency
Pitman-Moore Co., Indianapolis, Ind.	Novahistine Singlets, 100's	4/3/64	Label mix-up. One bottle contained Phenoxine Tabs
Southern Drug Mfg. Co.,[1,4] Knoxville, Tenn.	Novosol-Chemapley (triple sulfa)	4/6/64	Fails to disintegrate
E. R. Squibb & Sons, Brooklyn, N.Y.	Pentids 400	4/9/64	Product mix-up. 2 bottles each contained 1 Terfonyl Tab

/ Table 1: Lists of Drug Recalls

FIRM	PRODUCT	DATE	REASON
Merck Sharp & Dohme, West Point, Pa.	Dronactin 4's	4/23/64	Label mix-up. Some packets contained Phenergan
Upjohn Company, Kalamazoo, Mich.	Depo-Testosterone	4/30/64	Label mix-up. Outside carton bears wrong lot no.
Abbott Laboratories,[1,7] N. Chicago, Ill.	NaCL 0.9% Injection, 1000 cc	4/30/64	Label mix-up. Some bottles labeled as 5% Dextrose in Water
Kirkman Laboratories, Seattle, Wash.	Sodium Fluoride 1.0 mg	5/13/64	Cross-contamination with diethylstilbestrol
Ciba Pharmaceutical Co., Summit, N.J.	Ritalin 10 mg	5/13/64	Label mix-up. Labeled as Serpasil 0.25
E. R. Squibb & Sons, Brooklyn, N.Y.	Penicillin, Streptomycin	5/19/64	Printing error. Shows 400,00 units instead of 400,000 units
E. R. Squibb & Sons, Brooklyn, N.Y.	Stilbetin 5 mg Niacin 100 mg	5/20/64	Label mix-up. Bottles labeled Stilbetin contain niacin and vice versa
Morton Pharmaceuticals, Inc.,[1,7] Memphis, Tenn.	Pentaerythritol Tetranitrate Tabs	5/22/64	Excess potency

FIRM	PRODUCT	DATE	REASON
Nysco Labs, Inc.,[1,7] Long Island City, N.Y.	Triple Enzyme Tabs	6/2/64	Label mix-up. Rear panel labeled Triple Barbiturate Tabs
Chas. Pfizer & Co., New York, N.Y.	Tetracyn I.V. 250 mg & 500 mg	6/3/64	Contains pyrogens
Philadelphia Labs, Philadelphia, Pa.	Digoxin 0.25 mg tabs	6/8/64	Variation in potency. Potency ind. tabs vary 50%–240% of label declaration
Hamilton Pharmacal Co., Hamilton, N.Y.	Mastitis Ointment	6/22/64	Low potency. 33% of label declaration
Mallinckrodt Pharmaceuticals, St. Louis, Mo.	Conray 400 (Contrast Media) Na Iothalamate	6/22/64	Label mix-up. Immediate container labeled "Conray" (Meglumine Iothalamate) for which different dosage is required
E. R. Squibb & Sons,[1,7] Brooklyn, N.Y.	Digitoxin 0.2 mg tabs	6/23/64	Penicillin contamination
E. R. Squibb & Sons,[1,7] Brooklyn, N.Y.	Kenacort 4 mg tabs	6/23/64	Penicillin contamination

FIRM	PRODUCT	DATE	REASON
E. R. Squibb & Sons,[1,7] Brooklyn, N.Y.	Phenobarbital 30 mg tabs	6/23/64	Penicillin contamination
E. R. Squibb & Sons, Brooklyn, N.Y.	Mycostatin Tabs (vaginal)	6/23/64	Penicillin contamination
E. R. Squibb & Sons,[1,7] Brooklyn, N.Y.	Thiamine 100 mg tabs	6/23/64	Penicillin contamination
Masti-Kure Products Co., Norwich, Conn.	Mastitis Ointment	6/26/64	Low potency. 30.3% of labeled potency
Schering Corporation, Bloomfield, N.J.	Trilafon 16 mg	7/1/64	Label mix-up. Labeled as 8 mg
E. R. Squibb & Sons,[1,7] Brooklyn, N.Y.	Terfonyl	7/2/64	Penicillin contamination
E. R. Squibb & Sons,[1,7] Brooklyn, N.Y.	Kenacort 1 mg	7/2/64	Penicillin contamination
E. R. Squibb & Sons, Brooklyn, N.Y.	Sumycin 125 mg	7/2/64	Penicillin contamination
E. R. Squibb & Sons,[1,7] Brooklyn, N.Y.	Ascorbic Acid 500 mg	7/2/64	Penicillin contamination
E. R. Squibb & Sons, Brooklyn, N.Y.	Niacin 100 mg		Penicillin contamination
Rabin-Winters Corp., El Segundo, Calif.	Oil Eucalyptus	7/8/64	Label mix-up. Contains methyl salicylate

FIRM	PRODUCT	DATE	REASON
Philadelphia Labs, Philadelphia, Pa.	Digitoxin 0.1 mg	7/9/64	Variation in potency. Individual tablet variation 81.3 to 91.9% of potency
E. R. Squibb & Sons, Brooklyn, N.Y.	Chloral Hydrate Syrup	7/14/64	Contaminated with chlorobenzene
R. P. Scherer Corp., Detroit, Mich.	Chloral Hydrate Caps	7/14/64	Contaminated with chlorobenzene
Rabin-Winters Corp., El Segundo, Calif.	Tincture Arnica N.F.	7/15/64	Label mixup. Labeled as Oil Eucalyptus
E. R. Squibb & Sons,[1,7] Brooklyn, N.Y.	Kenacort 4 mg tabs	7/15/64	Penicillin contamination
E. R. Squibb & Sons,[1,7] Brooklyn, N.Y.	Kenacort 2 mg tabs	7/15/64	Penicillin contamination
E. R. Squibb & Sons, Brooklyn, N.Y.	Dicalcium Phosphate with Viosterol	7/15/64	Penicillin contamination
E. R. Squibb & Sons, Brooklyn, N.Y.	Naturetin 5 mg	7/15/64	Penicillin contamination
E. R. Squibb & Sons, Brooklyn, N.Y.	Milk of Magnesia Tabs	7/15/64	Penicillin contamination
Upjohn Company, Kalamazoo, Mich.	Tolbutamide	8/7/64	Label mixup

FIRM	PRODUCT	DATE	REASON
Masti-Kure Products Co.,[1,7] Norwich, Conn.	Mastitis Ointment	8/11/64	Subpotent in penicillin
Hamilton Pharmacal Co., Hamilton, N.Y.	Mastitis Ointment	8/11/64	Subpotent in penicillin
Abbott Laboratories,[1,7] N. Chicago, Ill.	Dextrose 10% Saline	8/13/64	Label mix-up. Labeled as Dextrose 2½% in Lactated Ringer Solution
Stanley Drug Prods., Inc., Portland, Ore.	Para Amino Salicylic Acid (PAS)	8/13/64	Contaminated with diethylstilbestrol
Cutter Labs, Inc., Chattanooga, Tenn.	Polysal "M"	8/13/64	Label mix-up. Polysal bottle when inverted reads Polysal "M"; labeled as Polysal when bottle is upright in use
Burrough Bros. Mfg. Co., Baltimore, Md.	Sodium Salicylate USP 0.32 gm	8/17/64	Failed USP test for disintegration
Abbott Laboratories,[1,7] N. Chicago, Ill.	Dextrose 5% in ½ normal saline	8/20/64	Label mix-up. Caps labeled Dextrose 5% in Saline

FIRM	PRODUCT	DATE	REASON
Abbott Laboratories, N. Chicago, Ill.	Various other batches of intravenous solutions recalled between August 19 and September 4, 1964, because of finding 1 to 6 mislabeled bottles per batch.		
Hamilton Pharmacal Co., Hamilton, N.Y.	Mastitis Ointment	8/26/64	Low potency Low penicillin
Masti-Kure Products Co.,[1,7] Norwich, Conn.	Mastitis Ointment	8/26/64	Low potency Low penicillin
Philadelphia Labs, Philadelphia, Pa.	APC #2 Green	9/8/64	Ingredient substitution. Acacia used in error for caffeine
Walker Laboratories, Mount Vernon, N.Y.	Quinamin+ Coricidin D (physician samples)	9/10/64	Label mix-up. Coricidin D samples labeled Quinamin
A. H. Robins Co., Richmond, Va.	Robitussin AC	9/11/64	Ingredient substitution. Brompheniramine substituted for pheniramine
Grant Chemical Co.,[1,7] Coudersport, Pa.	Epsom Salts USP	9/11/64	Label mix-up. Some packages contain boric acid
Lederle Laboratories, Pearl River, N.Y.	Achromycin V 100 mg	9/21/64	Label mix-up. Individual cartons labeled 250 mg

FIRM	PRODUCT	DATE	REASON
Chas. Pfizer & Co., New York, N.Y.	Penicillin 200,000 units	9/21/64	Product mixup. 250,-000 units found in one bottle
DuMont Pharmacal Co., Philadelphia, Pa.	Stilbestrol 0.5 mg	9/23/64	Label mixup
E. R. Squibb & Sons, Brooklyn, N.Y.	Mysteclin—F	9/29/64	Product mixup. One foreign capsule found
Philadelphia Labs, Philadelphia, Pa.	Buffered Penicillin G 250,000 units	10/6/64	Low potency
Hallmark Laboratories, Chicago, Ill.	Thiamine HCl 100 mg	10/6/64	Low potency
Vitamix Corporation, Philadelphia, Pa.	Hydrocortisone Acetate, aqueous suspension	10/1/64	Nonsterile
Merck Sharp & Dohme, Philadelphia, Pa.	Sulfasuxidine	10/5/64	Label mixup. Labeled as Sulfathalidine
Richlyn Labs, Inc., Philadelphia, Pa.	Estrogenic Substances	10/5/64	Low potency
Baxter Labs, Inc., Morton Grove, Ill.	Levugen 10% with Electrolyte #48	10/7/64	Label mixup. Labeled as Travert 10% in water
E. R. Squibb & Sons, New Brunswick, N.J.	Crysticillin 300,000 units	10/9/64	Label mixup. 20 vial cartons contained Distrycillin

FIRM	PRODUCT	DATE	REASON
Lloyd, Dabney & Westerfield, Inc., Cincinnati, Ohio	Dex-Cel-Ate	10/9/64	Ingredient substitution. d1-methamphetamine used in place of d-methamphetamine
Fellows Testagar, Detroit, Mich.	Estrone 2 mg/cc	10/9/64	Bacterial contamination
Delavan Company, Philadelphia, Pa.	d-desoxyephedrine 10 mg	10/12/64	Ingredient mixup. Contained didesoxyephedrine
Denver Serum Co., Denver, Colo.	Densulfa	10/15/64	Label mixup. Triple Sulfa 4% labeled as 8%
Chas. Pfizer & Co.,[1,7] New York, N.Y.	Terramycin Isojects 100 mg and 250 mg	10/16/64	Label mixup. Cartons containing 250 mg labeled as 100 mg
Chas. Pfizer & Co., New York, N.Y.	Penicillin 1,200,000 units	10/16/64	Label mixup. Penicillin in cartons labeled Streptomycin
Delta Laboratories, Inglewood, Calif.	Bovicil Mastitis Therapy	10/19/64	Label mixup. Syringe carton labeled Bovamycin

FIRM	PRODUCT	DATE	REASON
Zenith Labs., Inc., Englewood, N.J.	Theobromine and Phenobarbital Tabs	10/23/64	Penicillin contamination
Zenith Labs, Inc., Englewood, N.J.	Brewer's Yeast	10/23/64	Penicillin contamination
Zenith Labs, Inc., Englewood, N.J.	Meprobamate Tabs	10/23/64	Penicillin contamination
Zenith Labs, Inc., Englewood, N.J.	Reserpine Tabs	10/23/64	Penicillin contamination
Burrough Bros. Mfg. Co., Baltimore, Md.	Milk of Bismuth	10/28/64	Contaminated with bismuth sulfide
Upjohn Company, Kalamazoo, Mich.	Predef 2X Liquid	10/28/64	Low potency
Merck Sharp & Dohme, Philadelphia, Pa.	Cortone Acetate 0.5% ophthalmic suspension	10/27/64	Label mix-up. Labeled as Hydrocortone Acetate
Riders Ltd., Saugus, Calif.	Cortisone 25 mg	11/2/64	Low potency
Brewer & Co., Inc., Worcester, Mass.	Vancara Caps	11/9/64	Low potency
E. R. Squibb & Sons, New Brunswick, N.J.	Distrycillin	11/9/64	Label mix-up. Crysticillin labeled as Distrycillin
Chas. Pfizer & Co.,[1,7] New York, N.Y.	Procaine Penicillin Suspension	11/13/64	Nonsterile
E. R. Squibb & Sons, New York, N.Y.	Crysticillin 300 AS	12/1/64	Carton mix-up

FIRM	PRODUCT	DATE	REASON
Santa Pharmaceuticals, Buffalo, N.Y.	Marla Contact Lens Solution	11/30/64	Nonsterile
E. R. Squibb & Sons, New York, N.Y.	Streptomycin Injection	11/30/64	Penicillin contamination
E. R. Squibb & Sons, New York, N.Y.	Dihydrostreptomycin Injection	11/30/64	Penicillin contamination
E. Fougera & Co., New York, N.Y.	Chemestrogen 2 mg tabs	12/2/64	Label mix-up. Labeled as 5 mg tabs
E. Fougera & Co., New York, N.Y.	Genoscopalamine 0.5 mg tabs	12/2/64	Printing error. Labeled as 0.5 gm
Endo Labs, Inc., Garden City, N.Y.	Endolac Tabs	12/9/64	Subpotency
C. B. Fleet Co., Lynchburg, Va.	Theophylline rectal unit	12/9/64	Mold contamination
Wm. S. Merrell Co., Cincinnati, Ohio	Bentyl HCl 20 mg/2cc	12/9/64	Label mix-up. Labeled as codeine phosphate injection
Burrough Bros. Mfg. Co., Baltimore, Md.	Phenyl Salicylate Tabs	12/14/64	Improper disintegration
Bristol Laboratories, Syracuse, N.Y.	Tetrex APC Caps	12/15/64	Label mix-up. Polycillin Caps labeled as Tetrex
Parke, Davis & Co., Detroit, Mich.	Streptomycin	12/15/64	Penicillin contamination

/ Table 1: Lists of Drug Recalls

FIRM	PRODUCT	DATE	REASON
Norden Laboratories, Lincoln, Neb.	Sulfatose Injection 250 cc	12/22/64	Low potency
Geigy Chemical Corp., Ardsley, N.Y.	Dulcolax 5 mg tabs	12/18/64	Product mixup. Tofranil 10 mg tab found in Dulcolax bottle
Vent Air Contact Lens Specialists, New York, N.Y.	Vent Air Sterisoak and Cleansing Solution	12/28/64	Nonsterile
G. D. Searle & Co., Chicago, Ill.	Enovid	12/31/64	Label mix-up. 5 mg tab labeled as 2.5 mg
Lemmon Pharmacal Co., Sellersville, Pa.	Polycort Nasal Suspension	12/23/64	Low potency
Barry Labs, Inc., Detroit, Mich.	Progesterone 25 mg/cc vials	12/23/64	Excess potency

Drug Recalls (Requested or Voluntary), January 1 to December 31, 1963

FIRM	PRODUCT	DATE	REASON
Richlyn Labs, Inc., Philadelphia, Pa.	Heparin Sodium	1/11/63	Low potency. 67% of declared potency
Success Chemical Co., Brooklyn, N.Y.	Ferronvit Injection	1/30/63	Low potency. 40% in B_1, 10% in iron
Vitamin Corporation, Philadelphia, Pa.	Liver-Fol-B_{12} 10 cc vials	2/5/63	Low potency

FIRM	PRODUCT	DATE	REASON
Nysco Labs, Inc., Long Island City, N.Y.	Sinobel Nyscaps T.D. Caps	2/6/63	Ingredient substitution. Pyrilamine maleate subs. for pheniramine maleate
Robin Pharmacal Co., Brooklyn, N.Y.	Cotrin Tabs (cold tabs)	2/25/63	Low potency. Vit. C 80% deficient
Bolar Pharmaceutical Co., Brooklyn, N.Y.	Quinidine Sulfate 3 gr tabs	2/25/63	Low potency
Atlas Pharm. Labs, Inc., Detroit, Mich.	Hormone Injectables	3/5/63	Nonsterile
Vitarine Co., Inc., New York, N.Y.	Mensavite Tabs	3/8/63	Low potency
Nysco Labs, Inc., Long Island City, N.Y.	Duotrate with Phenobarbital	3/19/63	Label mix-up. Duotrate labels used on 2 or more bottles
Continental Pharmacal Co., Cleveland, Ohio	Lactated Ringers Solution	3/20/63	Pyrogen contamination
Continental Pharmacal Co., Cleveland, Ohio	Sodium Lactate Solution	3/28/63	Low potency. 46% deficient
E. R. Squibb & Sons, New York, N.Y.	Streptomycin Dimocillan RT	4/26/63	Label mix-up. Dimocillan vial in streptomycin carton

/ Table 1: Lists of Drug Recalls

FIRM	PRODUCT	DATE	REASON
Maurry Biological Co., Los Angeles, Calif.	Anematinic Injection (B_{12} liver folic acid)	4/29/63	Low potency. Deficiency in 2 of 3 active ingredients
Taylor Pharmacal Co., Decatur, Ill.	Calcium Gluconate Injectable—10 cc	4/30/63	Pyrogen contamination
Vitamix Corporation, Philadelphia, Pa.	Ergonovine Maleate Injectable	5/6/63	Low potency
Winning Peplow, Inc.,[1,7] Los Angeles, Calif.	Thyroid Tabs 1 gr	5/23/63	Excessive potency. Labeled as 1 gr; contain 2¾ gr
Lederle Laboratories, Pearl River, N.Y.	Delphicol Solution 16 oz	6/4/63	Ingredient mixup. Contaminated with N-Acetyl Kynex
Burrough Bros. Mfg. Co., Baltimore, Md.	Morphine Sulfate Tabs ¼ gr	6/19/63	Low potency. 70% deficient
E. R. Squibb & Sons, Brooklyn, N.Y.	Mycostatin Cream	6/27/63	Label mixup. Tubes of Mycostatin Cream in cartons labeled as Mycostatin Ointment
Robins Pharmacal Corp., New York, N.Y.	Reserpine 0.25 mg tabs	7/24/63	Low potency

FIRM	PRODUCT	DATE	REASON
Warner Labs, Inc., Brooklyn, N.Y.	Antispasmotic Tabs	7/29/63	Omission of ingredient. Label declares 16 mg phenobarbital whereas none present
Strong, Cobb & Co., Cleveland, Ohio	Copoietin Ferrous Tabs	8/2/63	Failure to disintegrate
International Distributors, Inc. (Plough, Inc.) Memphis, Tenn.	Castor Oil 1½ oz	8/5/63	Label mix-up. Some bottles labeled Gum Spirits of Turpentine
Richlyn Labs, Inc., Philadelphia, Pa.	Camphor Injection 30 cc	8/6/63	Label mix-up. Some vials contain Dipyrone
Barry Labs, Inc., Detroit, Mich.	Sodium Salicylate & Sodium I w/colchicine 20 cc	8/7/63	Ingredient error in Na Bisulfate & Colchicine
Lincoln Laboratories,[1,7] Decatur, Ill.	Stemutrolin Chorionic Gonadotropin	9/9/63	Low potency
Stanley Drug Prods., Inc., Portland, Ore.	Various vitamin preparations	9/17/63	Printing error in potency declarations
Invenex Pharmaceuticals, San Francisco, Calif.	Liver Injection 10 cc vials	9/20/63	Low potency. Mislabeled. End flap on box marked 20 mg/cc, main panel & vial marked 20 mcg/cc

/ *Table 1: Lists of Drug Recalls*

FIRM	PRODUCT	DATE	REASON
Burrough Bros. Mfg. Co., Baltimore, Md.	Atropine Sulfate 1/100 gr H.T.	9/20/63	Low potency. 75% of declared potency
Chas. Pfizer & Co., Brooklyn, N.Y.	Pot. Penicillin G-USP Tabs, 200,000 units	10/7/63	Label mix-up. Bottle labeled Pot. Pen. G contained Diabinase
Tablerock Laboratories, Greenville, S.C.	Trimerdi Tabs (triple sulfa)	10/30/63	Fails disintegration test
Maurry Biological Co., Los Angeles, Calif.	Chorionic Gonadotropin	12/5/63	Low potency. 25% of labeled potency
Penn Labs (White Cross), Philadelphia, Pa.	Hydrogen Peroxide 3 oz	12/9/63	Contaminated with propyl alcohol
McNeil Labs, Inc., Philadelphia, Pa.	Butabel RA Butaserpazide	12/17/63	Label mix-up. Butabel labeled as Butaserpazide
Ridlin Mfg. Co., Dallas, Texas	Isopropyl Alcohol 1 gallon	12/23/63	Label mix-up. Isopropyl alcohol labeled as acetone.

Drug Recalls (*Requested or Voluntary*), *October 1 to December 31, 1962*

Eli Lilly & Co., Indianapolis, Ind.	"Tycopan" Vitamin-Mineral Supplement	10/12/62	Label mixup

FIRM	PRODUCT	DATE	REASON
Morton Pharmaceuticals,[1,7] Memphis, Tenn.	Methyl Testosterone 10 mg tabs	10/15/62	Deficient in active ingredient
Geigy Pharmaceuticals, Yonkers, N.Y.	Persantin Injection (cardiac dilator)	10/26/62	Nonsterile
Chicago Pharmacal Co., Chicago, Ill.	Aplexal Injection	11/2/62	Deficient in vit. B_{12} and folic acid
Glenbrook Laboratories, Trenton, N.J.	Fletchers Aspir-aid for Children—Fletchers Cold Tabs for Children	11/14/62	Label mixup
E. R. Squibb & Sons, Brooklyn, N.Y.	Pentids Soluble (penicillin tabs)	12/5/62	Diethylstilbestrol tabs substituted for penicillin tabs (1 bottle)
Burrough Bros. Mfg. Co., Baltimore, Md.	NT Nitroglycerin tabs Fenadin Caps	12/20/62	Low potency. Product mixup. (NTN tabs). Quinine Sulfate Caps substituted for Fenadin
Rabin-Winters Corp.,[1,4] El Segundo, Calif.	Nicotinic Acid Tabs	12/26/62	Label mixup. Labeled as Vitamin C
Bolar Pharmaceutical Co., Brooklyn, N.Y.	Sulfadiazine, Aspirin Digoxin, Digitalis & Tripelennamine	12/27/62	Low potency (4 products)
Pennex Prod. Co., Pittsburgh, Pa.	Ascorbic Acid Tabs	12/31/62	Product mixup. Aspirin substituted

Actions Involving "Current Good Manufacturing Practice" Section Citation Cases

FIRM	CHARGES	PRESENT STATUS OF CASE
Scientific Chemical Co., Monrovia, Calif.	Medical diagnostic agents manufactured without satisfactory controls	Hearing held. Case placed in permanent abeyance by FDA's District office on March 4, 1964
The Stuart Company, Pasadena, Calif.	Sulfonamide drug mislabeled as a vitamin preparation	Hearing held. Case placed in permanent abeyance by FDA's District office on June 3, 1964
J. H. Bloch, Canton, Ohio	"Poho Oil" manufactured without satisfactory controls	Hearing held. Case placed in permanent abeyance by FDA's District office on May 27, 1964
Hampton Mfg. Co., Inc., New Rochelle, N.Y.	Adhesive bandages manufactured without satisfactory controls	Hearing held. Case placed in permanent abeyance by FDA's District office on Sept. 21, 1964
E. R. Squibb & Sons, New York, N.Y.	Various drugs manufactured without satisfactory controls	Hearing held. Case placed in permanent abeyance by FDA's headquarters on March 11, 1965
Abbott Laboratories, North Chicago, Ill.	Various drugs manufactured without satisfactory controls	Hearing held. Case placed in permanent abeyance by FDA's District office on March 16, 1965

FIRM	CHARGES	PRESENT STATUS OF CASE
Wyeth Laboratories, Philadelphia, Pa.	"Aludrox" manufactured without satisfactory controls	Hearing held. Case placed in permanent abeyance by FDA's District office on Dec. 1, 1964
Dixie Laboratories, Seagoville, Texas	Mineral oil repacked without satisfactory controls (contaminated by isopropyl alcohol)	Hearing held. Case placed in permanent abeyance by FDA's District office on Sept. 24, 1964
	Citrate of magnesia manufactured under improper conditions	Hearing held. Case placed in permanent abeyance by FDA's District office on May 13, 1965
Chas. Pfizer & Co., New York, N.Y.	Several drugs mislabeled because of inadequate controls	Hearing held. Case placed in permanent abeyance by FDA's District office on May 25, 1965
Kapco, Inc., Kalamazoo, Mich.	"Digesto" tablets manufactured under conditions not in keeping with current good manufacturing practices	Hearing held. Case placed in permanent abeyance by FDA's District office on June 10, 1965
Prosecution Cases		
Stanley Blackman Labs, South Hackensack, N.J.	Manufactured reserpine preparation without satisfactory controls	Case filed in Court. Defendant pleaded not guilty
Seizure Cases		
Dixie Laboratories, Seagoville, Texas	Mineral oil repacked without satisfactory controls (contaminated with isopropyl alcohol)	Product seized. Case closed by condemnation decree, July 14, 1964

/ Table 1: Lists of Drug Recalls

FIRM	CHARGES	PRESENT STATUS OF CASE
Zenith Labs, Inc., Englewood, N.J.	Hormone-vitamin preparation in tablet form, manufactured without satisfactory controls (tablets do not disintegrate properly)	Product seized. Case closed by condemnation decree, February 8, 1965
Zenith Labs, Inc., Englewood, N.J.	Amphetamine-barbiturate preparation in capsule form, manufactured without satisfactory controls (capsules are below potency)	Product seized. Case closed by condemnation decree, May 21, 1965
Biocraft Labs, Inc., East Paterson, N.J.	Ophthalmic ointment manufactured without satisfactory controls (contains metal particles)	Three products seized. Cases closed by condemnation decrees January 8, 20, and 27, 1965
Injunction Cases		
Continental Pharmacal Co., Cleveland, Ohio	Manufactured drugs without satisfactory controls	Injunction request filed with Court on August 12, 1963. Firm subsequently went out of business and the injunction request was withdrawn
Bolar Pharmaceutical Co., Brooklyn, N.Y.	Manufactured drugs without satisfactory controls	Injunction decree issued by Court on July 25, 1963. Still in effect
Drosnes-Lazenby Cancer Clinic, Pittsburgh, Pa. (Also known as Nutrition Service, Inc., Pittsburgh, Pa.)	Manufactured Mucorhicin (a drug intended for treating cancer) without satisfactory controls	Injunction decree issued by Court on February 17, 1964. Still in effect

FIRM	CHARGES	PRESENT STATUS OF CASE
Camall Company, Detroit, Mich.	Repacked drugs without satisfactory controls	Injunction decree issued by Court on October 1, 1964. Still in effect
Richlyn Labs, Inc., Philadelphia, Pa.	Manufactured drugs without satisfactory controls	Injunction decree issued by Court on October 9, 1964. Still in effect

List II

Drug Recalls (Requested or Voluntary), January 1 to June 30, 1965

FIRM	PRODUCT	DATE	REASON
Barry Labs, Inc.,[1,2] Detroit, Mich.	Bar-Gesterone	2/8/65	Bacterial contamination
Stanley Blackman Labs[1,2] (Westly Labs) S. Hackensack, N.J.	Quinine Sulfate NF XI	2/17/65	Product contains metal fragment, wood and paper
Ryson Labs, Inc., Orange, N.J.	Phenobarbital ½ gr	4/13/65	Label mixup and subpotent
Abbott Laboratories, N. Chicago, Ill.	Dextrose 5% in water	4/13/65	Defective caps, nonsterile
Arizona Labs, Inc., Phoenix, Ariz.	Apmix CT Tabs	4/19/65	Label mixup. Label declares 5 mg amphetamine, contains 15 mg
Smith, Miller & Patch, New Brunswick, N.J.	Duogen Suspension	4/23/65	Low potency
E. R. Squibb & Sons, New Brunswick, N.J.	Pot. Penicillin 200,000 units	4/23/65	Label mixup

FIRM	PRODUCT	DATE	REASON
Direct Labs, Inc., Buffalo, N.Y.	Liver Injection	4/26/65	Low potency
Success Chemical Co., Brooklyn, N.Y.	Kor-Val Nasal Inhaler	4/28/65	Substitution of dl-desoxyephedrine for d-desoxyephedrine
Picker X-ray Corp., White Plains, N.Y.	Dionisil	5/3/65	Penicillin contamination
Ayerst Laboratories, New York, N.Y.	Beminal Forte	4/30/65	Penicillin contamination
Ayerst Laboratories, New York, N.Y.	Bemotmic Caps	4/30/65	Penicillin contamination
Ayerst Laboratories, New York, N.Y.	Grisactin 125 mg	5/4/65	Penicillin contamination
Richlyn Labs, Inc., Philadelphia, Pa.	Tribarbital Tabs	5/4/65	Penicillin contamination
Richlyn Labs, Inc., Philadelphia, Pa.	Ascorbic Acid	5/4/65	Penicillin contamination
Physicians Products Co., Petersburg, Va.	Contramal Caps	5/7/65	Penicillin contamination
Wyeth Laboratories, Philadelphia, Pa.	Zactane Tabs	5/10/65	Penicillin contamination
Wyeth Laboratories, Philadelphia, Pa.	Spartase Tabs	5/10/65	Penicillin contamination

FIRM	PRODUCT	DATE	REASON
Wyeth Laboratories, Philadelphia, Pa.	Proketazine Tabs	5/10/65	Penicillin contamination
Parke, Davis & Co., Detroit, Mich.	Viomycin	5/10/65	Penicillin contamination
E. R. Squibb & Sons, New Brunswick, N.J.	Procaine Penicillin in aqueous suspension in disposable syringes	4/15/65	Particle size too large to eject
Franklin Serum Co., Denver, Colo.	CDM Solution 5% Dextrose	5/13/65	Low potency
Philadelphia Labs, Philadelphia, Pa.	DAS 10 mg tabs	5/14/65	Penicillin contamination
Ayerst Laboratories, New York, N.Y.	Hibitone Lozenges	5/14/65	Penicillin contamination
Ayerst Laboratories, New York, N.Y.	Maturon Tabs	5/14/65	Penicillin contamination
Wallace Laboratories, New York, N.Y.	Somocort Tabs	5/14/65	Penicillin contamination
White Labs, Inc., Kenilworth, N.J.	Disomer (Dexbrompheniramine maleate)	5/18/65	Low potency
Hoffmann-LaRoche, Inc., Nutley, N.J.	Valium (diazepam) dosage cards	5/20/65	Product mixup
S. J. Tutag & Co., Detroit, Mich.	Prednisolone Injection 50 mg	5/20/65	Nonsterile
S. J. Tutag & Co., Detroit, Mich.	Prednisolone Injection 25 mg	5/20/65	Nonsterile
Atlas Pharm. Co., Detroit, Mich.	Testosterone Injection 50 mg	5/20/65	Nonsterile

FIRM	PRODUCT	DATE	REASON
Atlas Pharm. Co., Detroit, Mich.	Testosterone 25 mg	5/24/65	Nonsterile
Baltimore Biological Labs, Baltimore, Md.	Toxo A Sensitivity Discs 08–466	5/24/65	Low potency
Abbott Laboratories, N. Chicago, Ill.	Erythromid Film-tabs	5/26/65	Penicillin contamination
Abbott Laboratories, N. Chicago, Ill.	Bacitracin Oph. Ointment ⅛ oz.	5/26/65	Low potency
McKesson Laboratories, Bridgeport, Conn.	Sulfa & Cream Tartar Lozenges	6/1/65	Penicillin contamination
McKesson Laboratories, Bridgeport, Conn.	Thiamine 50 mg tabs	6/1/65	Penicillin contamination
McKesson Laboratories, Bridgeport, Conn.	Soda Mint Tabs	6/1/65	Penicillin contamination
McKesson Laboratories, Bridgeport, Conn.	Children's Aspirin	6/1/65	Penicillin contamination
McKesson Laboratories, Bridgeport, Conn.	Meprobamate Tabs	6/1/65	Penicillin contamination
Approved Sales, Buffalo, N.Y.	Amphetamine Sulfate 10 mg tabs	6/3/65	Printing error
Philadelphia Labs, Philadelphia, Pa.	Apadex Tabs	6/14/65	Penicillin contamination
Lederle Laboratories, Pearl River, N.Y.	Neptazine 50 mg tabs	6/15/65	Penicillin contamination
Lederle Laboratories, Pearl River, N.Y.	Declomycin	6/15/65	Low potency
E. R. Squibb & Sons, New York, N.Y.	Kenalog-S	6/17/65	Low potency

FIRM	PRODUCT	DATE	REASON
Upjohn Company, Kalamazoo, Mich.	Deltasone (prednisone 5 mg)	6/22/65	Printing error
Premo Pharmacal Co., S. Hackensack, N.J.	Penazo Sulforin Tabs	6/30/65	Penicillin contamination
Premo Pharmacal Co., S. Hackensack, N.J.	Thyroid 2 gr tabs	6/30/65	Penicillin contamination
Premo Pharmacal Co., S. Hackensack, N.J.	Butabarbital ½ gr tabs	6/30/65	Penicillin contamination
Premo Pharmacal Co., S. Hackensack, N.J.	Butabarbital ¼ gr tabs	6/30/65	Penicillin contamination
Premo Pharmacal Co., S. Hackensack, N.J.	Theobromine & Phenobarbital Tabs	6/30/65	Penicillin contamination
Premo Pharmacal Co., S. Hackensack, N.J.	Meprobamate Tabs	6/30/65	Penicillin contamination
Premo Pharmacal Co., S. Hackensack, N.J.	Codeine Sulfate Tabs	6/30/65	Penicillin contamination
Premo Pharmacal Co., S. Hackensack, N.J.	Sweetner Tabs	6/30/65	Penicillin contamination
Premo Pharmacal Co., S. Hackensack, N.J.	Cortisone Acetate Tabs	6/30/65	Penicillin contamination
Premo Pharmacal Co., S. Hackensack, N.J.	Neomycin Sulfate Tabs	6/30/65	Penicillin contamination

/ Table 1: Lists of Drug Recalls

Drug Recalls (Requested or Voluntary), January 1 to December 31, 1964

FIRM	PRODUCT	DATE	REASON
Medical Chemical Corp.,[1,6] Chicago, Ill.	Testosterone Propionate 30 cc	3/18/64	Label mix-up. Labeled as Progesterone
Davis-Edwards Pharmacal Co.,[1,5] Bronx, N.Y.	Aspirin 5 gr enteric coated	4/24/64	Erratic disintegration time
Rabin-Winters Corp.,[1,5] El Segundo, Calif.	Tincture of Iodide	8/6/64	Label mix-up. Labeled as Tincture of Iodine
S. E. Massengill Co.,[1,6] Bristol, Tenn.	Ammonium Chloride 0.5 gm tabs	8/7/64	Slow disintegration
Brewer & Co., Inc.,[1,2] Worchester, Mass.	Reserpine 0.1 mg 0.25 mg	8/26/64	Tablet potency variation 41–200%

Drug Recalls (Requested or Voluntary), January 1 to December 31, 1963

FIRM	PRODUCT	DATE	REASON
C. M. Bundy Co.,[1,3] Cincinnati, Ohio	DaCosta Tabs	5/28/63	Low potency in nitroglycerin

Pending Cases Involving "Current Good Manufacturing Practice" Section

Citation Cases

FIRM	CHARGES	PRESENT STATUS OF CASE
Delta Laboratories, Inglewood, Cal.	Manufactured Penstrepcin (a veterinary drug) without satisfactory controls	Hearing held on September 18, 1964, and District placed case in temporary abeyance on October 19, 1964

FIRM	CHARGES	PRESENT STATUS OF CASE
Columbia Pharm. Corp., Freeport, N.Y.	Manufactured drugs without satisfactory controls (plus other violations)	Citation authorized April 21, 1965. Case is in District
Zenith Labs, Inc., Englewood, N.J.	Manufactured drugs without satisfactory controls (plus other violations)	Citation authorized May 18, 1965. Case is in District
Prosecution Cases		
Barry Labs, Inc., Detroit, Mich.	Manufactured drugs without satisfactory controls (plus other violations)	Prosecution recommendation sent to General Counsel on June 10, 1965
Lanpar Company, Dallas, Texas	Manufactured drugs without satisfactory controls (plus other violations)	Prosecution recommendation sent to General Counsel on June 23, 1965
Brewer & Co., Inc., Worcester, Mass.	Manufactured drugs without satisfactory controls (plus other violations)	Prosecution recommendation sent to General Counsel on July 19, 1965
C. M. Bundy Co., Indianapolis, Ind.	Manufactured drugs without satisfactory controls (plus other violations)	District's prosecution recommendation now under review at FDA's headquarters

Conclusion

It is not the intent of the *Handbook* to suggest specific guidelines for action by doctors. It is enough to present doctors with facts and expect that they will adequately govern themselves, for all members of the profession wish to make decisions which are in the best interests of their patients. However, one practice taught in medical school but all too frequently overlooked is seeing to it that patients know the name of any drug they must buy with the doctor's prescription. They have a right to know; it is an exceptional instance when the patient would be better off not knowing.

The antisubstitution laws which exist in most states to ensure that "the medical profession be left free to prescribe what it sees fit and that the public be assured that it gets what the doctor prescribed" can of course be used to cut two ways. A glance at the *Handbook* will enable the doctor to see what are the most expensive brands of a given drug, and should he wish to do so, he is free to specify on the prescription blank what brand or brands he does NOT wish to be dispensed. This may make some pharmacists unhappy, but the patient will be protected and that is what is really important. Most of the progressive pharmacists I know have responded by carrying a line of reliable basic generics, which enables them to fill prescriptions made out in this manner.

No single patient of mine who has been treated with a generic-equivalent drug has experienced anything but the effect which could be expected. I have been unable to observe in patients any difference whatever between the efficacy of generics and that of brand-name drugs, nor has there ever been a suggestion that the former are any more likely to cause untoward side effects.

So, for the reader who is a doctor: a reminder to instruct the pharmacist to label each prescription with the generic name of the drug. One need simply write the word "Label" on the prescription blank after the "Sig:"[34] and before the instructions to the patient.

For the reader who is a patient: when a doctor hands you

[34] See footnote 1, page 3.

a prescription, see whether it instructs the pharmacist to label and if it does not, ask the doctor please to do so. He will almost always be glad to, if only because it is a good safety practice to include it. The cost of drugs will begin to tumble only after it becomes common practice to label. If your prescription is one which will require frequent refills, you have a right to ask the druggist to obtain a supply of the drug when available from a reliable company whose price is reasonable. (The *Handbook* may be helpful in choosing one.) Should the druggist not like the idea, take your business to one who will cooperate; in a free enterprise system, competition works miracles.

Prescription Drug List

Here are listed names, sources, and prices of certain drugs. Those with names in capital letters are considered basic drugs. Others are listed because they are commonly used, but most if not all of these can usually be replaced by an equally effective, safe, less expensive basic drug.

The prices are those the druggist must pay (wholesale cost). While every effort was made to ensure against error in listing these prices, there is no guarantee. They have been taken from individual pharmaceutical company catalogues during 1966. Variation in dates of issuance of catalogues could account for some price differences. Companies reserve the right to change prices without notice. Indeed, changes may have occurred during preparation of the *Handbook*. In many cases, cost can be less than that listed if the druggist places more than a minimum order.

The list of manufacturers is not intended to be exhaustive.* The *Handbook* is not an advertising catalogue; no patronage is or will be accepted or solicited in any form or under any conditions. No specific product or company endorsement is implied. A company's record as determined by the frequency and nature of all of the drug recalls in which it has been involved (Table 1, pages 36–71, covers a thirty-three-month period only) and its acceptability as a bidder to the Defense Supply Agency of the United States government (Appendix A) are factors which physicians, patients, and pharmacists may wish to keep in mind. Obviously, a company's advertising budget is not necessarily a good criterion of its reliability.

The druggist's markup is usually 67 percent of the wholesale cost to show a profit of 40 percent of the retail price. An item which costs $3 is sold for $5. Most pharmacists maintain a "minimum prescription fee," a service charge, of from 50 cents to $2 but most commonly 75 cents or a dollar. The doctor, where it is practical and safe to do so, might wish to order as many doses of an inexpensive drug as will be covered by the minimum fee, especially if the drug is one which must be taken daily for a period of years. For example: if the doctor writes a prescription for digitoxin tablets, 0.1 milligram, an item which may cost the pharmacist as little as 20 cents per hundred, the patient might as well have a prescription ordering the dispensing of 300 tablets, if the druggist's markup is 67 percent and his minimum fee is $1.

All drugs listed here are prescription items. Most of them are included in either the *United States Pharmacopeia* or *The National Formulary*, as indicated by the initials following their names. This is not a treatise on pharmacology and there is absolutely no intention to imply that the information can be used to

* Drug manufacturers are listed here under shortened versions of their names. Most of these are listed under their full names in Appendix A (pages 160–67) or Appendix B (pages 168–70).

enable self-treatment. Physicians will recognize at once that the discussion of pharmacology is largely superficial; the *Handbook* is designed to be used in conjunction with an authoritative textbook of pharmacology, such as *The Pharmacological Basis of Therapeutics* by L. S. Goodman and A. Z. Gilman (New York, Macmillan, 1965).

It is assumed that all readers will wish to use the *Handbook* as a reference source of drug costs and that lay persons will be able to understand most of the discussion which it contains. However, here and there are statements which will probably have meaning to doctors alone.

*Contents**

* Drugs in capital letters are the *Handbook's* "basic" drugs, i.e., those which suffice for treating 90 percent or more of adult patients, treated by general practitioners or internists in the United States, who are not sick enough to be hospitalized.

I. Drugs Used in Infectious Disease

THE PENICILLINS, NATURAL AND SYNTHETIC

The pioneer and still the antibiotic combining highest therapeutic effectiveness with greatest all-round safety is common penicillin G. This was the first important member of a series of naturally occurring substances produced by various bacteria and fungi to become widely used in treating infections. Penicillin was introduced to everyday clinical medicine in 1942, although its discovery (or intimation of its existence) harks back to 1929 when a then obscure British bacteriologist, Alexander Fleming, working with the common germ staphylococcus, noticed that this germ failed to grow on a gelatinous, nutrient-impregnated surface immediately surrounding sites where colonies of the common fungus penicillium were growing. The fungus was present by accident; contamination of such culture plates is common because mold spores are present in the atmosphere and often settle on the gelatin surface if the cover is taken off for a few moments. Fleming appreciated the possible significance of the chance discovery that a growing colony of common penicillium mold can inhibit growth of a ubiquitous germ that is often the cause of serious disease. Surmising that the mold might be diffusing a chemical growth-inhibitory for bacteria through the gelatin in a concentric ring about the colony, he purposely turned to growing penicillium in large amounts, made crude filtered extracts of many combined colonies, and applied the material superficially to infected wounds. Patients were available for the purpose, since Fleming maintained his laboratory within St. Mary's, a large London hospital.

Results of Fleming's experiments on the possible therapeutic value of penicillium extract were not encouraging; we now know, thirty-six years later, that his extraction procedure was faulty. However, he described all of his findings in a journal which is customarily read at regular intervals by bacteriologists and other interested professionals. (It is only through the medium of books and journals that scientists and physicians all over the world can stay abreast of interesting current discoveries; all disciplined laboratory workers are expected to write up their most recent experiments and to read the reputable journals regularly.) So it was that many thoughtful persons, including Howard Florey, another British research physician, knew of Fleming's findings and kept them in mind. Ten years later, Florey and laboratory colleagues undertook to check and if possible to extend Fleming's discovery. They embarked on a systematic screening process to discover how many and what kinds of living organisms in addition to molds might be capable of inhibiting growth of other unrelated microorganisms. Fleming's original observations were easily confirmed, and using better extraction techniques Florey and his colleagues succeeded in making a crude material which when injected into mice prevented death from experimentally induced infection with the microorganism which commonly causes serious pneumonia in humans. Organic chemists set to work to isolate the pure ingredient responsible for the extract's activity and came up with a minuscule quantity of a substance later to be called "penicillin," which by good fortune turned out to be extremely toxic to germs but hardly at all to humans, except for those few who are allergic to it.

With the outbreak of World War II the potential military usefulness of penicillin in treating contaminated wounds and other infections was appreciated by all scientists. However, means for isolating the drug in large quantities were nonexistent, and the assistance of the pharmaceutical industry was solicited both in this country and in Britain. In the end, it was the publicly supported Northern Regional Research Laboratory of the United States Department of Agriculture in Peoria, Illinois, which found the means to produce penicillin cheaply and in massive quantities. This initial penicillin was named penicillin G—still its official, generic name—and it is still the preferred form of the drug for most purposes.

Penicillin G is, therefore, an unpatented therapeutic agent whose production within the United States is now accomplished by at least six corporations and in Europe by numerous others. Some concerns have had the temerity to advertise the drug by a catchy brand name and to charge a high price for it. The few doctors who have been taken in by this promotion are wasting their patients' money, for *by law* every batch of penicillin (or any other antibiotic, for that matter) intended for sale in the United States, whether manufactured here or abroad, must be laboratory tested and/or approved (i.e. "certified") by the Food and Drug Administration of the United States government. Thus, the least costly penicillin and all other antibiotics, no matter where produced, can be prescribed and used with assurance that they meet the *United States Pharmacopeia*'s standards of quality, purity, and potency. There is no reason for prescribing these substances by brand name when a generic equivalent is available.

POTASSIUM PENICILLIN G TABLETS, U.S.P. (buffered)

This is the basic and the most important of the penicillins. Readily absorbed from the gastrointestinal tract, it is the equivalent of any other oral penicillin preparation in terms of clinical effectiveness. Where particularly high blood levels are desired, the dose may be increased from the usual 3 tablets per day (at least one half hour before mealtime and at least two hours after having last eaten) to as many as 4 tablets three or four times per day. The major contraindication to its use is known allergy to penicillin. The great advantages of penicillin G are its low toxicity and its reasonable cost.

200,000 unit tablet (125 mgm)	#100	$1.25	Allen Pharm.
		1.00	Am. Quinine
		1.30	Carroll
		1.15	Columbia Med.
		1.75	Corvit
		1.45	Daniels
		1.62	Horton & Converse
		1.50	Lannett
		4.77	Lilly
		6.72*	Parke, Davis
		1.80	Penhurst
		.92	Pennex
		2.00	Pfizer
		1.35	Rondex
		6.62	Squibb (Pentids®-200)
		1.55	Supreme
		1.90	Towne, Paulsen
		1.35	Vita-Fore
		1.70	West-ward
		1.72	Wyeth

* 250,000 unit tablet

POTASSIUM PENICILLIN G TABLETS, U.S.P. (soluble)

A tablet or two dissolved in milk or fruit drink, Coca-cola, or ginger ale makes an excellent and inexpensive dosage form for children, feeble persons, and others who for any reason cannot swallow tablets. Be sure the tablet goes completely into solution and that the patient swallows it right away at a time when the stomach is empty. To make sure that the patient gets the complete dose, a little more liquid should be poured into the tumbler to pick up any remaining drug.

200,000 unit tablet (125 mgm)	#100	$1.62	Allen Pharm.
		1.10	Am. Quinine
		1.30	Carroll
		1.30	Columbia Med.
		1.95	Daniels
		1.70	Lannett
		6.72*	Lilly
		2.10	Penhurst
		1.55	Rondex
		1.75†	Supreme
		1.75	Vita-Fore
		1.80	West-ward

Note: The price for soluble penicillin G powder with a soluble buffer and flavor added ready for solution in water is $1.35 to the druggist for a bottle containing only 16 doses of 200,000 units each (Pentids® for Syrup [Squibb]). A disadvantage is that once in solution the antibiotic slowly loses its potency over a period of weeks, though not to a significant extent for at least two weeks. The tablets are stable indefinitely.

Several semisynthetic penicillins with narrow antibacterial spectra are now fortunately available for the treatment of infections due to "penicillin-resistant" (i.e. penicillinase-producing) strains of staphylococcus, and this is ordinarily their only use.

* 250,000 unit tablet
† Effervescent

Most of these infections develop in hospitalized patients, less frequently in ambulatory, nonhospitalized persons. (Many strains of the common and ubiquitous staphylococcus residing in and on hospital personnel and patients are by now resistant to penicillin G.) Therefore, penicillin G remains the agent of choice for treatment of mild localized staphylococcal infections in nonhospitalized patients. For more severe infections both penicillin G and one of the semisynthetic penicillins should be given together in case culture and sensitivity studies determine that the organism is resistant to penicillin G. Reason for using both is that, paradoxically, penicillin G, milligram for milligram, is a more potent antibiotic for eradicating staphylococci that can still be destroyed by it. As with penicillin G, the semisynthetic penicillins should be taken when the stomach has been without food for about two hours and at least half an hour before eating. Only preparations for oral use are listed below, but preparations for parenteral use (i.e. by injection) are available.

SODIUM OXACILLIN, U.S.P.

500 mgm capsule	#100	$34.29*	Bristol Labs (Prostaphlin®)
		32.93	Squibb (Resistopen®)

cloxacillin

250 mgm capsule		14.65	Bristol Labs (Tegopen®)

The recommended initial dose (*New Drugs*, 1966) is 500 milligrams four times daily for mildly and moderately ill patients, more for severely ill.

nafcillin

250 mgm capsules	#100	$25.50†	Wyeth (Unipen®)

Before the advent of chemotherapy and antibiotics, mild or moderate staphylococcal infections in ambulatory patients (most

* Actual listing $16.46/48
† Actual listing $6.12/24

commonly superficial infections in the form of skin abscesses, carbuncles, and impetigo) responded satisfactorily to proper hygiene and local application of heat. Inexpensive penicillin G is satisfactory for treatment in the vast majority of patients outside of hospitals. Not every ambulatory patient with such infections requires culture and sensitivity studies of pus or exudate (even if available, and often it is not). It is sensible to instruct the patient in the use of lots of soap and water, frequent changes of clean clothes and bedclothes, and local application of heat in any form, to caution him against squeezing the area, and to start penicillin G therapy in more than very mild and localized infections elsewhere than about the head and face. Only if no satisfactory improvement occurs after three or four days is it sensible to prescribe a substance as expensive as the semisynthetic penicillins. This is good public health practice, too, for who is to say that staphylococcus might not eventually develop resistance to the semisynthetics?

Note: Infections of the head and face warrant especially close attention and probably both types of penicillin for a start. A culture should be made of appropriate material and sensitivity tests performed.

AMPICILLIN

A broad-spectrum, penicillin-like semisynthetic which is especially useful in urinary tract infection where *Proteus* of certain kinds are the offending organism. It is not effective against penicillinase-producing staphylococcus, however. An excellent drug, expensive but well worth the price where indicated. *Allergic reactions to ampicillin are common (more than 10 percent of patients receiving it) and they can be very severe!*

250 mgm capsule	#100	$27.35	Bristol Labs (Polycillin®)
		27.36	Ayerst Labs (Penbritin®)
		27.50*	Wyeth (Omnipen®)

* Actual listing $6.60/24

TETRACYCLINES AND CONGENERS

The original "tetracyclines" were the chlor- and oxy-derivatives (marketed as Aureomycin ® and Terramycin ®), but their use has largely been supplanted by tetracycline, because it has been claimed that the latter is less likely to cause stomach upset than chlortetracycline. However, the difference if any is small. Within the year 1967 the patents will run out on Aureomycin® and Terramycin®, both of which can be expected to become available as inexpensive generics. This is fortunate, because the domestic production of generic tetracycline has been severely limited—a story too complicated for discussion here.

One other derivative, demethylchlortetracycline (marketed as Declomycin®), is less well excreted in the urine than tetracycline. Thus smaller doses may be given in order to achieve a given blood level. But this drug is more toxic than tetracycline in at least one respect: it more commonly causes sensitivity to sunlight, extensive blistering burns having necessitated hospitalization of some people taking it. Poor urinary excretion contraindicates use of the demethylchlor- derivative for urinary tract infections.

TETRACYCLINE HYDROCHLORIDE, U.S.P.

The workhorse of the broad-spectrum antibiotics.

250 mgm capsule	#100	$11.22	Lederle (Achromycin®)
		14.94	Upjohn (Panmycin®)
		14.96	Pfizer (Tetracyn®)
		14.95	Squibb (Steclin®)

Many drugstores and wholesalers have stocked large supplies of generic tetracycline manufactured by either domestic or foreign laboratories. In all cases the material must by law have been inspected and certified by the FDA.

The Department of Defense has on hand a supply of tetracycline manufactured at a cost of less than one cent per 250 milligram capsule by Rachel Laboratories of California.

tetracycline phosphate

No significant advantage over tetracycline hydrochloride.

250 mgm capsule	#100	$14.94	Upjohn (Panmycin Phosphate®)
		14.95	Bristol Labs (Tetrex®)
		14.95	Squibb (Sumycin®)

Chlortetracycline Hydrochloride, N.F.

Physicians should know that the patent on chlortetracycline will expire in 1967. It will then become available inexpensively as a generic, and for all practical purposes can be used interchangeably with tetracycline.

250 mgm capsule	#100	$11.22	Lederle (Aureomycin®)

Oxytetracycline, N.F.

250 mgm capsule		17.80	Pfizer (Terramycin®)

The comments about chlortetracycline apply equally well here.

Demethylchlortetracycline Hydrochloride, N.F.

150 mgm capsule	#100	$16.83	Lederle (Declomycin®)

Demethylchlortetracycline is expensive and is still available only by costly brand name. There is a widespread tendency on the part of physicians to prescribe it wherever "virus pneumonia" is suspected. This is because a certain percentage of "virus pneumonias" are not due to a virus at all but to a recently identified infectious organism called "Eaton Agent" (*Mycoplasma pneumoniae*). This organism is sensitive to both demethylchlortetracycline and tetracycline, and the latter (prescribed as a generic) is the agent of choice (less toxic, less expensive).

SULFONAMIDES AND DRUGS USED MAINLY FOR URINARY TRACT INFECTION

The discovery of the antibacterial effect of sulfonamide drugs constitutes another of the many fascinating chapters in pharmacology. The great Paul Ehrlich, a German microbiologist, had spent the latter part of the nineteenth century studying the ability of certain dyestuffs to make chemical attachments to tissues. By exposing living and dead tissues to various dyestuffs and studying them under the microscope, he discovered that dyes selectively stain certain parts of cells only. By exposing tissues to two or more dyes, he made it easy to distinguish the different parts of cells. Ehrlich was able to carry out his studies because the German organic dye industry was the most advanced in the world; he had easy access to many of its products. The ability of dyes to make firm chemical attachment to components of living tissue and to the substance of such naturally occurring materials as wool, cotton, and silk stimulated speculation that a dyestuff might be found which would selectively attach itself to and kill germs without doing harm to the human body. Various scientists, mostly European, made systematic searches for such agents during the early years of this century. One "azo" dye, harmless to humans who excrete it in the urine, was marketed in 1914 for use as a urinary antiseptic. Actually the drug is next to useless, although it may have a psychological effect because it colors the urine orange. (This has not deterred one pharmaceutical firm with a large advertising budget from selling this simple old-fashioned dyestuff under a brand name for a wholesale price of $48 per thousand 0.1 gram tablets. They are not rash enough to designate it a urinary "antiseptic," preferring to call it a "urinary analgesic." Imagine how difficult it must be to establish proof of such action! In any event, the same dye is available elsewhere by its generic name, phenazopyridine, for less than one third of $48!) In 1932, industrial chemists in Germany synthesized prontosil, another in a long line of azo dyestuffs. In 1935 this dye came to be tested by Gerhard Domagk, who was engaged in systematically testing dyestuffs for possible antibacterial activity. Prontosil was discovered to be effective in preventing death in mice injected with the common pneumonia organism. When this observation was published, research workers at the Pasteur Institute in Paris took up a study of prontosil and demonstrated that only one part of the prontosil molecule was necessary for the antibacterial activity; this was sulfanilamide. Since then many useful sulfonamide drugs have been synthesized, more effective and less toxic than sulfanilamide.

Sulfonamides are now used relatively rarely, having been supplanted for the most part by antibiotic drugs. (Sulfonamides are spoken of as *chemotherapeutic agents* rather than as *antibiotics*, the latter term being reserved for drugs produced by living microorganisms.) There is one notable exception, however. In the treatment of urinary tract infections sulfisoxazole, a highly soluble and relatively nontoxic sulfonamide, is usually the drug of choice. (Urinary tract infection not severe enough to require hospitalization but persisting—criterion: urine culture, *not* a simple urinalysis—after two to three weeks of sulfisoxazole treatment requires further investigation to determine the proper therapeutic agent.)

The comparatively recently released sulfonamides, advertised as advantageous by virtue of slower excretion, sulfadimethoxine (Madribon®) and sulfamethoxypyridazine (Kynex® and Midicel®) are more likely than sulfisoxazole to cause serious toxicity (Stevens-Johnson syndrome), enough so that warnings were sent this year to all physicians by the distributors of these drugs, which are not listed in the *Handbook*. Nor does the *Handbook* list sulfamethoxazole (Gantanol®), more expensive than sulfisoxazole but not superior. The addition of an azo dye to a sulfonamide is of dubious value and adds very considerably to cost.

SULFISOXAZOLE, U.S.P.

0.5 gm tablet	#1000	$17.50	Allen Pharm.
		12.00	Am. Quinine
		13.50	Carroll
		12.95	Columbia Med.
		14.50	Kasar
		13.80	Lannett
		16.95	Penhurst
		17.75	Pennex
		25.30	Roche (Gantrisin®)
		13.45	Rondex
		17.50	Stayner
		19.75	Towne, Paulsen
		21.54	U.S. Vitamin (Entusul®)
		11.95	Vita-Fore
		15.13	Vitarine
		18.00	West-ward

Since the most commonly prescribed adult daily dose of sulfisoxazole is eight 0.5 gram tablets per day, the daily cost to the patient can vary from 16 to 36 cents. The price spread is not as great here as with many drugs, but savings by buying the generic are considerable if the patient requires several weeks of continuous therapy, as many do.

Nitrofurantoin, U.S.P.

Used exclusively for treatment of urinary tract infection. Since most such infections are due to sulfonamide-sensitive *Escherichia coli*, sulfisoxazole is preferred to start treatment. Nitrofurantoin, a patented product, is very expensive.

100 mgm tablet	#100	$29.00	Eaton Labs (Furadantin®)

Average recommended dose in adults with acute urinary tract infection is 4 tablets per day.

AMPICILLIN (See page 87)

METHENAMINE MANDELATE, U.S.P.

One of the most rational methods of supplying prophylaxis in persons prone to develop recurrent urinary tract infection is by prescribing this official *U.S.P.* drug. The usual adult dose is 1 gram four times a day; this often suffices to acidify the urine while releasing a suppressive concentration of formaldehyde and a germ-killing concentration of un-ionized mandelic acid. Bacteria do not become resistant. It is essential that the urine be acidified to a pH at least as low as 5.0 and so it may be necessary to give an additional urine-acidifying agent—4 grams of ascorbic acid per day will do the trick at a cost of about 15 cents.

0.5 gm tablet	#1000	$12.00	Am. Quinine
		11.40	Carroll
		13.50	Daniels
		12.95	Penhurst
		12.00	Supreme
		15.00	Towne, Paulsen
		7.95	Vita-Fore
		29.15	Warner-Chilcott (Mandelamine®)
		15.70	West-ward

Note: This drug should never be given at the same time as the sulfonamide sulfamethizole (Thiosulfil®).

ANTITUBERCULOSIS DRUGS

ISONIAZID, U.S.P.

The discovery that the inexpensive, easily synthesized organic chemical isoniazid (INH) is a powerful but relatively nontoxic antituberculosis drug which can be taken by mouth was one of the most important scientific achievements of our time. As with most other pharmacological discoveries, the usefulness of isoniazid was determined by a combination of chance and educated guessing. INH is the keystone in tuberculosis therapy, supported by streptomycin (which must be injected) and another simple organic chemical called PAS (see below).

Since treatment is nearly always long-term, it is worth while and convenient to prescribe and purchase isoniazid in large quantities.

100 mgm tablet	#1000	$ 4.50	Allen Pharm.
		2.50	Am. Quinine
		4.95	Carroll
		3.85	Columbia Med.
		5.00	Corvit
		4.50	Daniels
		5.50	Horton & Converse
		3.00	Kasar
		11.40	Lilly
		4.85	Merrell (Tyvid®)
		3.40	Panray
		7.98	Parke, Davis (Niconyl®)
		4.95	Penhurst
		4.50	Rondex
		8.00	Squibb (Nydrazid®)
		4.75	Supreme
		5.75	Towne, Paulsen
		3.50	Vita-Fore
		5.44	Vitarine
		5.60	West-ward

AMINOSALICYLIC ACID, U.S.P. (Para-aminosalicylic Acid, PAS)

The original trial of PAS as an antituberculosis drug was undertaken because a basic science investigator had noted that it suppressed growth and multiplication of tubercle bacilli in the test tube. The reasons leading to its trial in this regard are simple and logical but beyond the scope of the *Handbook*. The drug is an old-fashioned chemical known for many years to all organic chemists, although its usefulness in medicine was not known until 1946.

500 mgm tablet	#1000	$ 8.00	Allen Pharm.
		5.00	Am. Quinine
		6.50	Carroll
		6.25	Columbia Med.
		7.20	Daniels
		7.75	Kasar
		6.60	Lannett
		15.15	Lilly
		8.40	Merrell
		5.35	Panray
		6.40	Penhurst
		7.20	Rondex
		5.75	Vita-Fore

There is a slight price difference depending upon whether tablets are coated or not.

Since both isoniazid and PAS had been on the shelves of organic chemistry laboratories long before anyone suspected their medical usefulness, neither is patented. However, this has not deterred some companies from selling them under brand names—precisely the kind of confusion which many in the medical profession would like to dispel.

ANTIFUNGUS DRUGS

GRISEOFULVIN, U.S.P.

An antibiotic with the ability to combat certain common fungus infections of hair, skin, and nails which until recently were untreatable in any satisfactory way. However, this is still a relatively new drug and until more is known of its toxicity it seems wise to avoid using it for trivial infections. It is at present the only drug which may produce some improvement in severe fungus infection of nails and nail beds.

125 mgm tablet (ultra-fine crystals allegedly allowing more efficient absorption and higher blood levels)	#100	$6.50*	Schering (Fulvicin®)
		6.20	McNeil (Grifulvin®)
		6.56	Ayerst Labs (Grisactin®)

One month is the minimum recommended duration of treatment, but in some cases treatment may have to continue for a year and total retail cost will be about $95.

TOLNAFTATE

A new preparation for treating fungus infections of the skin. Many cases of "athlete's foot" clear dramatically in a few days.

1% solution for topical application	10 cc	$1.98	Schering (Tinactin®)
1% cream for topical application	15 gm tube	1.94	Schering (Tinactin®)

candicidin

For treatment of infection due to the fungus *Candida albicans*, an infection most commonly referred to as "thrush."

0.06% ointment	75 gm tube	$2.70	Schmid (Candeptin®)
tablet for vaginal insertion	#28	3.90	Schmid (Candeptin®)

* Actual listing $3.90/60

NYSTATIN, U.S.P.

For treatment of "thrush."

500,000 unit tablet for systemic administration	#100	$8.82	Squibb (Mycostatin®)
Cream ointment for topical treatment, 100,000 units/gm	15 gm tube	1.26	Squibb (Mycostatin®)
100,000 unit vaginal tablet	#15	1.26	Squibb (Mycostatin®)

ANTIPROTOZOAN DRUGS

The two following drugs are used within the United States mainly as adjuncts in treatment of rheumatoid arthritis and of discoid lupus erythematosus, and are given as prophylactics to travelers to parts of the world where susceptible strains of malaria are endemic.

CHLOROQUINE PHOSPHATE, U.S.P.

250 mgm tablet	#100	$2.80	Allen Pharm.
		3.50	Carroll
		2.15	Columbia Med.
		3.00	West-ward
		6.70	Winthrop (Aralen®)

hydroxychloroquine phosphate

Same uses as chloroquine phosphate.

200 mgm tablet	#100	$7.35	Winthrop (Plaquenil®)

Note: Long-term treatment (many months or years) with both chloroquine and hydrochloroquine has been reported in some few cases to be accompanied by development of irreversible visual abnormalities, even blindness, so careful observation of the patient is indicated while on either of these drugs.

METRONIDAZOLE

For treatment of infection due to trichomonads, one-celled creatures which are a common cause of vaginal itch and discharge. Males frequently harbor the organism in the urethra, so sexual partners ought to be treated at the same time.

250 mgm tablet	#60*	$8.40	Searle (Flagyl®)
500 mgm tablet for vaginal insertion	#10	2.88	Searle (Flagyl®)

MISCELLANEOUS

The three antibiotics listed below are frequently prescribed, too often without good reason.

Chloramphenicol, U.S.P.

The first broad-spectrum antibiotic (1947) which could be taken orally (streptomycin [1943] must be injected), and a powerful one. However, its toxicity is potentially so grave that it is not recommended for use in nonhospitalized patients. If it is so used, arrangements should be made to examine the patient's blood every other day. Its only indications for use are: typhoid fever, rare Rickettsia infections, and urinary tract infections due to organisms resistant to other antibiotics. It should not be prescribed for any other purposes. Tetracycline, sulfonamides, and streptomycin, alone or in combination, will substitute for the other uses of chloramphenicol.

250 mgm capsule	#100	$30.60	Parke, Davis (Chloromycetin®)
		6.60	West-ward

Note: The patent on chloramphenicol has now expired (October 1966).

* For ten-day course of treatment for sexual partners.

Erythromycin, U.S.P. (and several salts)

The major indication for use is where there is known allergy to penicillin. The spectrum of activity is about the same as that of penicillin. Toxicity is rarely a serious problem with erythromycin (except as noted), but cost is a good deal more than that of penicillin.

erythromycin ethylsuccinate

200 mgm chewable tablet	#100	$18.00*	Abbott (Erythrocin®)

Erythromycin Stearate, U.S.P.

100 mgm tablet	9.96	Abbott (Erythrocin® Film-tab)
250 mgm tablet	21.99	"

Erythromycin (crystalline), U.S.P.

100 mgm tablet	9.96	Lilly (Ilotycin®)
250 mgm tablet	21.99	"
100 mgm tablet	9.96	Upjohn
250 mgm tablet	21.99	"

erythromycin estolate

125 mgm capsule	11.91	Lilly (Ilosone®)
250 mgm capsule	21.99	"
125 mgm chewable tablet	12.12†	"

Note: Erythromycin estolate may cause jaundice. Advantage over other erythromycin oral preparations: less destruction by stomach acid.

* Actual listing $9.00/50
† Actual listing $6.06/50

Phenoxymethyl Penicillin, N.F., and Potassium Phenoxymethyl Penicillin, U.S.P. (both usually called "penicillin V")

Because of greater resistance to gastric acid, this form of penicillin, unlike penicillin G, may be given with or after meals, an expensive luxury. (See pages 84–85.) The general range of effectiveness and incidence of allergic reactions are similar to those of orally administered penicillin G. Penicillin V is not yet available as a generic marketed without a brand name.

The parenteral use of penicillin G (i.e. by injection) is still the initial treatment of choice in severe infections caused by hemolytic streptococci, pneumococci, gonococci, and susceptible staphylococci. *Penicillin V is no more effective than penicillin G against the penicillin-resistant staphylococcus and therefore cannot substitute for the semisynthetic penicillins on page 86.*

125 mgm* chewable wafer	#50	$4.27	Abbott (Compocillin V®)
125 mgm capsule	#50	4.50	Lilly (V-Cillin®)
125 mgm tablet	#36	3.24	Wyeth (Pen-Vee® Oral)

Note: The advertising claim is made (and is undoubtedly correct) that three or four 200,000 unit penicillin G tablets would have to be taken to achieve the same concentration of active drug in the blood as can be achieved with a single 200,000 unit tablet of penicillin V if the drugs are taken at mealtimes. Advertisements cannot point out, however, that 800,000 units of penicillin G in tablet form need cost only about half as much as 200,000 units of penicillin V.

* Equivalent to 200,000 units penicillin G

II. Sedatives and Drugs for Sleep

SEDATIVES (SO-CALLED "TRANQUILIZERS")

PHENOBARBITAL, U.S.P. (See also Drugs for Sleep)

Phenobarbital, one of the oldest of the barbiturates, when given in small doses remains the "tranquilizer" of choice for most anxious patients treated by the internist and general practitioner. Like other sedatives, phenobarbital can be addicting if taken in large enough amounts over a long period; its withdrawal can cause typical delirium tremens and convulsions. Similar symptoms have now been described following administration and discontinuation of meprobamate (Equanil®, Miltown®), chlordiazepoxide (Librium®), and diazepam (Valium®).

One disadvantage of phenobarbital is its power. Since barbiturates are the most powerful of the sedatives, the suicidal patient may find it easier to kill himself with an overdose of phenobarbital than with some other agents. However, a patient who is thought to be suicidal belongs in the hospital under close observation.

Phenobarbital is inexpensive and universally available. The wholesale cost of a thousand 15 milligram tablets runs from about 50 cents to a dollar. Since many druggists maintain a minimum prescription price, a patient will frequently find himself paying up to $2 for 50 or fewer 15 milligram tablets, an amount which may cost the druggist 5 cents or less. In spite of this, the drug is much less expensive than other sedatives.

Note: Experts in behavioral pharmacology find no major differences in the effects on animal behavior of small doses of phenobarbital and those caused by the so-called "minor tranquilizers," such as meprobamate and chlordiazepoxide.

CHLORAL HYDRATE, U.S.P.

500 mgm capsules	#100	$1.62	Allen Pharm.
		2.00	Am. Quinine

1.60	Carroll
1.20	Columbia Med.
1.50	Daniels
10.70*	Kasar
1.60	Lannett
4.20	Merck Sharp & Dohme (Somnos®)
1.55	Penhurst
1.40	Pennex
1.55	Rondex
4.20	Squibb (Noctec®)
2.00	Stayner
1.60	Supreme
2.15	Towne, Paulsen
1.35	Vita-Fore
1.70	Vitarine
1.70	West-ward

Chloral hydrate, one of the oldest and safest sedatives, excellent as a "tranquilizer" during the day (500 mgm every three to six hours) and as a sleep inducer in larger doses, is available in capsule form from a large number of distributors at a cost to the patient which need not exceed 2 cents per dose.

Many of these same distributors sell the drug in liquid form. One gallon contains approximately 800 teaspoonsful. A few examples:

CHLORAL HYDRATE SYRUP, U.S.P.

1 gallon (500 mgm/tsp)	$ 5.95	Carroll
	8.00	Rondex
	12.95	Squibb (Noctec®)
	8.35	West-ward

Here cost to the druggist can be as little as eight tenths of a cent per 500 milligrams. This dose should not cost the patient more than 1.5 cents.

* Price for 1000 capsules

Mallinckrodt Chemical Works sells 450 grams of U.S.P. grade chloral hydrate crystals for $2.69. Where medication is being supplied to a population at public expense, institutional dispensaries should give serious consideration to making up their own chloral hydrate syrup.

Few substances have been advertised as widely to the medical profession as sedatives. Public relations divisions of major drug manufacturers have succeeded nicely in getting both the public and physicians (including many pharmacologists) to adopt the term "tranquilizer" as if there were really an obvious and measurable difference in the clinical effect of such substances as meprobamate, chlordiazepoxide, and a host of others as compared to that of phenobarbital or chloral hydrate when used in sedative doses. It is particularly disturbing to note (see below) the frequency with which sedatives are marketed with trade names which are designed to sell. This promotional method has effectively influenced many physicians and much of the public. The following are frequently prescribed sedatives not defined as basic drugs by the *Handbook*.

Chlordiazepoxide Hydrochloride, N.F.

10 mgm capsule #100 $7.00* Roche (Librium®)

Meprobamate, N.F.

400 mgm tablet	3.50	Allen Pharm.
	3.15	Carroll
	3.40	Columbia Med.
	3.80	Lannett
	3.35	Penhurst
	3.10	Pennex
	3.25	Rondex
	4.00	Stayner

* Actual listing $3.50/50

		3.95	Towne, Paulsen
		6.50	Wallace Labs (Miltown®)
		3.80	West-ward
		5.80	Wyeth (Equanil®)

chlormezanone

100 mgm tablet	#100	$7.00	Winthrop (Trancopal®)

diazepam

5 mgm tablet	8.00*	Roche (Valium®)

emylcamate

200 mgm tablet	5.94	Merck Sharp & Dohme (Striatran®)

hydroxyphenamate

200 mgm tablet	8.50†	Armour (Listica®)

mephenoxalone

400 mgm tablet	5.80‡	Lakeside (Lenetran®)
	5.80§	Lederle (Trepidone®)

oxanamide

400 mgm tablet	9.00‖	Merrell (Quiactin®)

oxazepam

15 mgm tablet	5.60	Wyeth (Serax®)

* Actual listing $4.00/50
† Actual listing $4.25/50
‡ Actual listing $2.90/50
§ Actual listing $2.90/50
‖ Actual listing $4.50/50

phenaglycodol			
200 mgm tablet	#100	$4.20	Lilly (Ultran®)
tybamate			
250 mgm tablet		7.44	Wallace Labs (Solacen®)
Hydroxyzine Hydrochloride, N.F.			
25 mgm tablet		6.97	Roerig (Atarax®)
hydroxyzine pamoate			
25 mgm tablet		6.97	Pfizer (Vistaril®)
buclizine			
25 mgm tablet		5.57	Stuart (Softran®)
benactyzine hydrochloride			
1 mgm tablet		3.60	Merck Sharp & Dohme (Suavitil®)
ectylurea			
300 mgm tablet		7.26*	Upjohn (Levanil®)

DRUGS FOR SLEEP (HYPNOTICS)

Any sedative in large enough dose will serve as a "sleeping pill." Phenobarbital, 30 to 60 milligrams, remains an excellent hypnotic. The quicker-acting barbiturates, secobarbital and pentobarbital, are more frequently prescribed for this purpose, however. Chloral hydrate in a 1 to 2 gram dose is an effective

* Actual listing $3.63/50

hypnotic for most patients, especially the elderly. For those who find barbiturates or chloral hydrate unsatisfactory, there are some nonbarbiturate sedatives which are good hypnotics.

PHENOBARBITAL, U.S.P.

The usual dose is 1 or 2 tablets. The effect lasts about eight hours.

30 mgm tablet	#1000	approx. $.65 up to $1.25	Many manufacturers

SODIUM PENTOBARBITAL, U.S.P.

Begins to act within thirty minutes, and effect lasts about six hours.

100 mgm capsule	#1000	$16.20	Abbott (Nembutal®)
		6.00	Am. Quinine
		5.35	Carroll
		5.05	Columbia Med.
		5.40	Daniels
		6.00	Horton & Converse
		5.00	Kasar
		5.60	Lannett
		20.22*	Lilly
		4.50	Penhurst
		5.50	Pennex
		4.95	Rondex
		5.75	Supreme
		7.65	Towne, Paulsen
		3.95	Vita-Fore
		6.46	Vitarine
		7.40	West-ward

Pentobarbital is one of the best examples of a drug that is widely sold by a large number of distributors under its generic

* Actual listing $10.11/500

name. While the prices shown above apply to 100 milligram *capsules*, many companies will supply it at considerably less cost as *tablets*. It is equally effective in either form.

SODIUM SECOBARBITAL, U.S.P.

Begins to act in about fifteen minutes and effect lasts three to six hours.

100 mgm capsule	#1000	$ 6.20	Am. Quinine
		6.25	Carroll
		5.25	Columbia Med.
		7.20	Daniels
		4.50	Kasar
		6.20	Lannett
		18.30*	Lilly (Seconal®)
		5.95	Panray
		6.50	Penhurst
		6.20	Pennex
		5.25	Rondex
		8.75	Stayner
		6.96	Supreme
		7.85	Towne, Paulsen
		4.95	Vita-Fore
		7.31	Vitarine
		8.60	West-ward

CHLORAL HYDRATE, U.S.P. (See pages 101–3)

Glutethimide, N.F.

0.5 gm tablet	#1000	$37.60	CIBA (Doriden®)

Methyprylon, N.F.

200 mgm tablet		44.00†	Roche (Noludar®)

* Actual listing $9.15/500
† Actual listing $22.00/500

Advertisements for the last two drugs emphasize that they are "not barbiturates," which must not be interpreted to mean that these drugs have inherent advantages over barbiturates. Both glutethimide and methyprylon lend themselves in excessive usage or dosage to the very same abuses as barbiturates—habituation, addiction, and suicide! "Tolerance" to their effect develops just as it does to barbiturates.

III. Appetite Suppressants (Anorexiants)

DEXTROAMPHETAMINE SULFATE, U.S.P.

5 mgm tablet	#1000	$ 2.00	Allen Pharm.
		1.00	Am. Quinine
		1.50	Carroll
		1.35	Columbia Med.
		2.45	Daniels
		1.60	Horton & Converse
		1.15	Kasar
		1.48	Lannett
		1.50	Penhurst
		1.50	Pennex
		1.95	Rondex
		22.60*	Smith Kline & French (Dexedrine®)
		2.25	Supreme
		3.50	Towne, Paulsen
		1.25	Vita-Fore
		1.70	Vitarine
		2.00	West-ward

Dextroamphetamine causes nervousness, sleeplessness, and other stimulatory effects as well as curbing appetite. There are several other related synthetic derivatives which are advertised as appetite suppressants:

* "Spansules" cost $2.80 per 50 ($56.00/1000).

benzphetamine hydrochloride

50 mgm tablet	#1000	$41.70	Upjohn (Didrex®)

chlorphentermine hydrochloride

65 mgm tablet		103.50	Warner-Chilcott (Pre-Sate®)

diethylpropion hydrochloride

25 mgm tablet		43.40	Merrell (Tenuate®)

phendimetrazine bitartrate

35 mgm tablet		40.02	Ayerst Labs (Plegine®)

Phenmetrazine Hydrochloride, N.F.

25 mgm tablet		41.55	Geigy (Preludin®)

phentermine resin

15 mgm capsule		100.20*	Strasenburgh (Ionamin®)

phentermine hydrochloride

8 mgm tablet		35.00	Dorsey Labs (Wilpo®)

Most of these have only recently appeared on the market, and it is still much too early to accept without reservation advertising claims that any one is relatively more of an appetite suppressant while less of a stimulant than dextroamphetamine. In fact, experts on this class of drugs are skeptical of such claims. The one of the group which has been on the market longest (phenmetrazine, introduced in 1958) has already been subject to abuse by persons taking it for its central stimulant effects. The result in some instances has been a psychotic illness with behaviorial abnormalities including hallucinations and delusions (*New*

* Actual listing $40.08/400

Drugs, 1966). The same has long been known to occur with excessive use of dextroamphetamine.

A regimen effective in most patients who need an anorexiant, one which remains very inexpensive, is: dextroamphetamine, 5 milligrams about three hours before what is usually the largest daily meal, plus phenobarbital, 15 milligrams. The patient, provided he is reliable, is instructed to use the phenobarbital in sufficient amount just to cancel out "jitters" or sleeplessness if they are bothersome. In most people appetite suppression occurs only when there is also some degree of central nervous system stimulation, and sometimes more than 5 milligrams of dextroamphetamine is required to achieve this.

dextroamphetamine-amobarbital combinations

Widely prescribed are tablets and timed-disintegration capsules containing combinations of dextroamphetamine and amobarbital, a barbiturate whose action is akin to that of phenobarbital although its duration of action may be a little less long. The *Handbook* has already committed itself to the opinion that the prescription of combinations of drugs in a single tablet or capsule is generally not preferred practice, but it is recognized that many responsible and competent physicians might hold a different view in selected cases. In instances where patient or physician prefers a combination, the following information on availability and cost may be of interest:

tablet, 5 mgm	#1000	$ 2.48	Am. Quinine
dextroamphetamine		4.80	Daniels
plus approx. 30		4.00	Lannett
mgm amobarbital		3.60	Penhurst
		2.75	Rondex
		24.85	Smith Kline & French (Dexamyl®)
		5.80	West-ward

timed-disintegration capsule, 10 mgm dextroamphetamine plus approx. 60 mgm amobarbital	#1000	$ 9.00	Allen Pharm.
		10.50	Carroll
		9.25	Columbia Med.
		11.50	Daniels
		12.60	Lannett
		11.95	Penhurst
		9.75	Pennex
		8.95	Rondex
		68.56	Smith Kline & French (Dexamyl® Spansule No. 1)
		10.50	Supreme
		9.00	Vita-Fore
		11.90	Vitarine
		15.85	West-ward
timed-disintegration capsule, 15 mgm dextroamphetamine plus 90–100 mgm amobarbital		10.80	Allen Pharm.
		11.75	Carroll
		9.95	Columbia Med.
		12.50	Daniels
		14.00	Lannett
		14.95	Penhurst
		9.95	Rondex
		86.62	Smith Kline & French (Dexamyl® Spansule No. 2)
		12.00	Supreme
		10.00	Vita-Fore
		12.75	Vitarine
		18.15	West-ward

IV. Anti-Epilepsy Drug

SODIUM DIPHENYLHYDANTOIN, U.S.P.

A happy result of basic chemical studies, this drug is related structurally to phenobarbital but is more anticonvulsant and less sedative. Its introduction into clinical medicine in 1938 was a milestone; tens of thousands of persons with epilepsy are able to lead nearly normal lives because of it.

0.1 gm capsule	#1000	$ 8.75	Consolidated Midland
		8.50	Corvit
		8.00	Horton & Converse
		10.08	Parke, Davis (Dilantin®)
		6.95	Penhurst
		6.95	Raway
		6.38	Vitarine
		7.30	West-ward

The recognition that phenobarbital, too, has this property was similarly a milestone and antedates this discovery.

V. Antinausea Drugs

Nausea is usually a short-lived symptom, self-limited, commonly due to chemically induced inflammation of the stomach or intestine, as from excessive alcohol intake or irritation caused by infection. The nauseated person wishes to be left alone to sleep or doze until he feels better. Disturbance in the form of noise or jostling may provoke vomiting. While many patients need nothing but quiet bed rest, if a drug is required a safe sedative is the agent of choice. Phenobarbital, 15 or 30 milligrams, is a good treatment for mild nausea. For more serious nausea or vomiting, one of the antinauseants listed below may be helpful. Persistent unexplained nausea or vomiting is reason for hospitalization.

ANTIHISTAMINES WITH STRONG ANTINAUSEA AND ANTI-MOTION-SICKNESS EFFECT

DIPHENHYDRAMINE HYDROCHLORIDE, U.S.P.

A good and inexpensive antinauseant. (See Antihistamines, page 118, for cost.)

buclizine hydrochloride

25 mgm tablet	#100	$5.57	Stuart (Softran®)

Cyclizine Hydrochloride, U.S.P.

50 mgm tablet		3.30	Burroughs Wellcome (Marezine®)

Meclizine Hydrochloride, U.S.P.

25 mgm tablet		6.12	Pfizer (Bonine®)

Meclizine has recently been alleged to cause birth defects when given to pregnant laboratory animals. Therefore, it and chemically related cyclizine (Marezine®) and chlorcyclizine (Perazil®) ought not to be given to women who have any reason to believe that nausea might be an early sign of pregnancy.

PHENOTHIAZINES

PROMETHAZINE HYDROCHLORIDE, U.S.P.

A useful substance, chemically a phenothiazine, promethazine has powerful sedative, antinausea, anti-motion-sickness, and antihistamine properties.

25 mgm tablet	#100	$5.73	Wyeth (Phenergan®)
25 mgm suppository	#12	1.88	Wyeth (Phenergan®)

Other phenothiazines commonly used as antinauseants (but *not* as anti-motion-sickness drugs) are probably less safe. They are:

Chlorpromazine Hydrochloride, U.S.P.

25 mgm tablet	#100	$6.06	Smith Kline & French (Thorazine®)

100 mgm suppository	#6	$1.53	Smith Kline & French (Thorazine®)

Chlorpromazine is the only drug listed in the *U.S.P.* as a "tranquilizer." In very large doses it is much used in mental hospitals for the purpose of quieting agitated psychotic patients, and is very effective.

Prochlorperazine Maleate, U.S.P.

10 mgm tablet	#100	$7.86	Smith Kline & French (Compazine®)
25 mgm suppository	#6	1.53	Smith Kline & French (Compazine®)

Promazine Hydrochloride, N.F.

25 mgm tablet	#50	2.91	Wyeth (Sparine®)

The toxic effects of phenothiazines include severe fall in blood pressure, acute neurological symptoms (excepting promethazine), jaundice due to small bile-duct obstruction (excepting promethazine), agranulocytosis (depressed manufacture of white blood cells), and skin reactions.

The antinauseant effects of this class of compounds are often striking and beneficial, but their prescription for the usual case of self-limited gastrointestinal disturbance is questionable in view of their well-documented toxicity. They are *not* useful in the nausea and vomiting of vestibular-apparatus disturbance, e.g. motion sickness (except for promethazine), and are contraindicated for nausea of early pregnancy. (Not because they have ever been shown to cause birth defects, but because prudence tells us that at this very critical period the developing embryo is best protected from any and all unnecessary chemical influences.)

VI. Pain Relievers (Analgesics)

ASPIRIN, U.S.P.

Aspirin, manufactured into tablets by a large variety of firms and available without prescription, can be expensive or inexpensive depending upon the extent to which the buyer has been previously influenced by high-priced advertising. Many pharmaceutical manufacturers make a "soft" aspirin, one that breaks up quickly in the stomach. This has the advantage of causing less localized irritation. Your druggist will know of several large reliable firms that manufacture reasonably priced aspirin tablets.

All of the aspirin powder manufactured in the United States comes from six sources: Rexall Chemical Company, Dow Chemical Company, Miles Laboratories, Inc., Monsanto Company, Norwich Pharmacal Company, and Sterling Drug, Inc.

0.3 gm tablet	#1000	approx. $1.00	Many manufacturers

PROPOXYPHENE HYDROCHLORIDE, U.S.P.

65 mgm capsule	#100	$7.02	Lilly (Darvon®)
65 mgm capsule plus aspirin, phenacetin, and caffeine		7.32	Lilly (Darvon® Compound)

CODEINE SULFATE, N.F.

The manufacture and sale of this narcotic substance and also its price are rigidly dictated by the United States government: 450 grams costs approximately $350. Thus, a single 15 milligram tablet has wholesale value of approximately one cent. A representative price to druggists is $11.80 per thousand 15 milligram tablets (Vitarine). The *Handbook* lists Codeine Sulfate, N.F., rather than Codeine Phosphate, U.S.P., because the latter, being more soluble, is more bitter to the taste.

VII. Antihistamines

The physician is constantly bombarded with new antihistamine agents because it is relatively simple to synthesize new patentable ones. This is so because a wide variety of organic compounds of the following general structure where X is carbon, oxygen, or nitrogen are likely to be antihistamines. The R's stand for any of a variety of organic chemical groups.

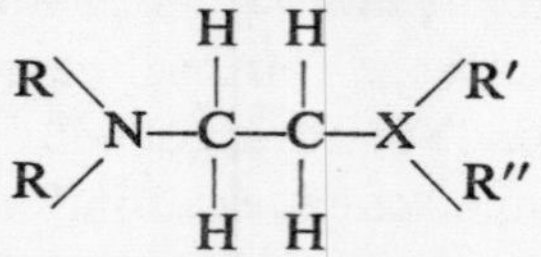

```
          H  H
R\        |  |     /R'
   N—C—C—X
R/        |  |     \R"
          H  H
```

Antihistamines are used in clinical medicine as much for their atropine-like and sedative side effects (and some for anti-motion-sickness and antinausea side effects) as they are for their actual antihistamine effect. While the ability to antagonize histamine is easily demonstrable in laboratory tests with certain animal species and in special experimental setups involving isolated organs and parts of organs, it is not so easily demonstrable in the human species, where very large doses have to be given by mouth in order to achieve a sufficiently high concentration in peripheral tissues to be effective. Yet even the recommended doses do cause obvious side effects. Thus, in mild seasonal hay fever, runny and stuffy nose may be alleviated but this may be due in part to the atropine-like side effect which inhibits glandular mucus secretion. Antihistamines are usually not effective in alleviating bronchospasm of asthma. Although it is probable that antihistamines are helpful in treating hives, it is hard to say so for certain, as hives is usually a transient, self-limited phenomenon. Thus, the subsidence of hives following administration of an antihistamine cannot necessarily be interpreted as the effect of the drug.

One frequent misuse of antihistamines in clinical medicine is their indiscriminate prescription for itch from whatever cause. While possibly helpful in itch associated with hives, antihistamines are probably not beneficial in other circumstances. Itch is pain in the skin and responds as pain elsewhere to analgesics, aspirin and codeine. This is most strikingly apparent in the morbid itch of chicken pox and that accompanying insect bites, in burns including sunburns, and in poison ivy where there are painful ("itchy") turgid vesicles. Administration of an antihistamine may help a little by virtue of its sedative effect, but there are more effective sedatives in the form of barbiturates and chloral hydrate.

There are three major classes of antihistamine drugs based on variations in chemical structure. One of the best known and oldest prototypes of each is given here, since it is impractical as well as unnecessary to list all, of which there are probably more than fifty. Furthermore, there are always advantages, aside from cost, in drawing attention to older and well-tried agents in any family of drugs.

CHLORPHENIRAMINE MALEATE, U.S.P.

Very potent as an antihistamine, this agent is less likely to cause drowsiness than some others, although there is a great deal of individual variation. It is not a good antinauseant and is not effective against motion sickness.

4 mgm tablet	#1000	$ 6.00	Allen Pharm.
		2.00	Am. Quinine
		3.95	Carroll
		1.95	Columbia Med.
		4.50	Corvit
		5.60	Lannett
		3.70	Panray
		4.95	Penhurst
		20.59	Schering (Chlor-Trimeton®)
		4.10	Stanlabs
		1.95	Vita-Fore
		6.65	West-ward

DIPHENHYDRAMINE HYDROCHLORIDE, U.S.P.

Actions include a pronounced tendency to cause somnolence, which can be dangerous to those driving automobiles or working with heavy machinery. Gastrointestinal side effects are usually not marked. Diphenhydramine is effective against motion sickness and in this respect is the active principle in dimenhydrinate (see note below).

25 mgm capsule	#1000	$ 6.25	Columbia Med.
		4.75	Kasar
		7.00	Lannett
		12.84	Parke, Davis (Benadryl®)
		8.95	Penhurst
		5.95	Vita-Fore

Note: The anti-motion-sickness drug, dimenhydrinate (sold as Dramamine®), is simply a molecular combination of diphenhydramine and chlorotheophylline in which the active ingredient is the former. Since almost half of the weight of the combination is made up of the chlorotheophylline, the dose of dimenhydrinate which is equieffective with 25 milligrams of diphenhydramine hydrochloride is about 50 milligrams. Diphenhydramine hydrochloride is much less costly.

Dimenhydrinate, U.S.P.

50 mgm tablet	#1000	$36.00	Searle (Dramamine®)

TRIPELENNAMINE HYDROCHLORIDE, U.S.P.

A very good antihistamine. Likely to be less sedative than diphenhydramine but more likely to cause gastrointestinal upset. Not a good antinauseant and ineffective for motion sickness.

50 mgm tablet	#1000	$ 7.00	Allen Pharm.
		26.60	CIBA (Pyribenzamine®)
		4.35	Columbia Med.
		10.80	Horton & Converse
		4.75	Kasar
		9.80	Lannett
		9.50	Penhurst
		9.95	Rondex
		9.90	Stayner
		9.69	Vitarine
		9.70	West-ward

VIII. Drugs Which Suppress Cough (Antitussives)

CODEINE SULFATE, N.F.

The production of the powder, its price, and its sale to drug manufacturers are carefully controlled by the federal government because codeine is a narcotic. The bulk chemical costs approximately $350 for 450 grams. Therefore, the wholesale value of the codeine in a single 15 milligram tablet—the most frequently dispensed dosage form—is a little more than one cent. A representative price to druggists is $11.80 per thousand 15 milligram tablets (Vitarine).

Dextromethorphan Hydrobromide, N.F. (d-methorphan)

Any over-the-counter cough syrup containing this substance (look at the label) can be expected to have mild antitussive activity. No prescription is needed to purchase such medications. The danger in self-medication of cough which persists is obvious; so-called "cigarette cough" can be one of the most serious of symptoms and is reason to see a physician.

IX. Drugs for Asthma, or Bronchospasm (Bronchodilators)

AMINOPHYLLINE, U.S.P.

This drug is a molecular combination of theophylline with ethylenediamine. The latter is inert, but its presence increases the solubility of theophylline about twentyfold and this makes it possible to achieve effective blood levels of aminophylline when given by mouth. Contrary to widespread belief, oral administration of aminophylline, up to 100 milligrams four times daily (with meals and at bedtime), rarely causes nausea and many patients can take up to 200 milligrams each time. It is effective and can be inexpensive.

100 mgm tablet	#1000	$3.00	Allen Pharm.
		2.00	Am. Quinine
		2.20	Carroll
		2.05	Columbia Med.
		3.00	Corvit
		2.60	Daniels
		3.80	Horton & Converse
		2.20	Lannett
		2.10	Panray
		2.35	Penhurst
		3.00	Pennex
		2.45	Rondex
		8.16	Searle
		3.60	Stayner
		2.61	Supreme
		2.25	U.S. Vitamin
		2.25	Vita-Fore
		2.45	Vitarine
		3.40	West-ward

EPHEDRINE SULFATE, U.S.P.

The structure of ephedrine is enough like that of epinephrine for it to have many of the latter's effects, of which one is bronchodilation. While these effects are less intense than those produced by epinephrine, they last for hours rather than minutes. The reason for this lengthy action is that ephedrine is not broken down in the body. This is not true of epinephrine, which is rapidly destroyed. Isolated in pure form in 1885, ephedrine is the active principle of mahuang, a Chinese herb medicine known for centuries.

25 mgm capsule	#1000	$ 5.40	Allen Pharm.
		4.20	Am. Quinine
		4.50	Carroll
		4.95	Columbia Med.
		5.00	Corvit
		5.75	Horton & Converse
		4.25	Kasar
		4.00	Lannett
		10.80	Lilly
		12.00	Parke, Davis
		5.85	Penhurst
		6.30	Pennex
		4.75	Rondex
		5.00	Supreme
		5.95	Vita-Fore
		2.82	Vitarine
		6.45	West-ward

theophylline-ephedrine-phenobarbital combination

tablet, 130 mgm theophylline, 24 mgm ephedrine, 8 mgm phenobarbital	7.95	Allen Pharm.
	5.25	Carroll
	4.95	Columbia Med.
	7.95	Daniels
	4.65	Horton & Converse
	3.50	Kasar
	5.60	Lannett
	4.30	Panray

		8.95	Supreme
		24.00	Warner-Chilcott (Tedral®)
		7.35	West-ward

aminophylline-ephedrine-phenobarbital combination

This combination can be expected to be more useful to some people than theophylline-ephedrine-phenobarbital.

tablet, 130 mgm aminophylline, 15 mgm ephedrine, 15 mgm phenobarbital	#1000	$4.80	Carroll

If the pharmacist has none in stock, 100 milligrams aminophylline, 25 milligrams ephedrine sulfate, plus 15 milligrams phenobarbital can be prescribed individually.

ADRENAL STEROIDS (See Section XIV, pages 143–46)

X. Topical Nasal Decongestant

According to the president of one small, reliable drug-manufacturing concern, "the cost of making up phenylephrine nose drops is a joke." The ingredients in a gallon of 1 percent phenylephrine solution (including buffer solutions and preservative) cost the manufacturer approximately $3.50.

The patient probably ought not to buy more than an ounce of the solution at a time, because it comes in a dropper bottle and when he puts the tip of the dropper into his nose he contaminates it with myriad bacteria and molds. When the dropper cap is put back on the bottle, the organisms multiply in the fluid and within a few days particulate material representing colonies of bacteria and molds can be seen in the bottle when it is held up to the light. This is the point at which to discard the bottle. (It goes without saying that one should not use nose drops which have already been used by someone else.) The solution is always marketed in a brown bottle, for exposure to light accelerates decomposition of phenylephrine. A yellow or pink tint indicates oxidation (and inactivation).

Phenylephrine is available over the counter (i.e. without a prescription) in one-ounce bottles (.25 percent concentration) at a retail price of between 75 cents and one dollar. This means that a gallon of material with ingredients worth less than $5 is ultimately sold at a retail price of as much as $120!

PHENYLEPHRINE HYDROCHLORIDE, U.S.P.

0.25% solution for nose drops	450 cc	$2.00	Carroll
(0.5% and 1% solutions also	(1 pint)	1.50	Columbia Med.
available)		1.75	Daniels
		1.20	Lannett
		1.95	Penhurst
		1.60	Pennex
		1.75	Rondex
		2.04	Vitarine
		5.76	Winthrop (Neo-Synephrine®)

Other kinds of vasoconstrictor nose drops are available, all related chemically to phenylephrine. Therefore all of them, if used in excess, could make the blood pressure rise. Furthermore, most others have more inherent ability to cause fast or irregular heart action than phenylephrine. (Physicians will recognize phenylephrine as a sympathomimetic agent with very strong "alpha-receptor" stimulating effect and little ability to stimulate the rate-increasing "beta-receptors" in the heart.)

XI. Drugs for High Blood Pressure (Antihypertension Drugs)

The modern treatment of high blood pressure (of unknown cause) with drugs is as much an art as a science. Several effective agents are now available and the trick is to find the proper one or combination which best suits a particular patient. They are discussed below roughly in order of increasing power (which is the order in which they are usually prescribed).

RESERPINE, U.S.P.

The introduction of reserpine within the past fifteen years represents an important advance. There are several substances in the plant *Rauwolfia serpentina* which can lower the blood pressure; the most potent of them is reserpine, now available as a pure, inexpensive compound. The single domestic manufacturer listed by the Federal Trade Commission (1964), is S. B. Penick & Company of New York. As the drug has a cumulative effect, 0.1 milligram per day is usually a sufficient dose for the ambulatory patient. In this dosage serious toxic side effects (the most serious being severe mental depression) are unlikely. Reserpine may cause blood pressure to fall by depleting the sympathetic side of the autonomic nervous system and certain brain centers of chemical transmitter substance (norepinephrine), but this has by no means been established as fact.

0.1 mgm tablet	#1000	$ 1.60	Allen Pharm.
		1.30	Am. Quinine
		1.25	Carroll
		23.50	CIBA (Serpasil®)
		1.10	Columbia Med.
		2.00	Corvit
		1.30	Daniels
		1.75	Horton & Converse

	1.40	Kasar
	1.80	Lannett
	7.80	Lilly (Sandril®)
	1.90	Panray (Serpanray®)
	1.35	Penhurst
	1.25	Pennex
	1.30	Rondex
	2.50	Stayner
	1.43	Supreme
	2.75	Towne, Paulsen
	19.98	Upjohn (Reserpoid®)
	.70	Vita-Fore
	1.77	Vitarine
	2.00	West-ward

Some widely advertised reserpine-like drugs are listed below. Reserpine can be substituted for any of them.

alseroxylon fraction of rauwolfia serpentina

2 mgm tablet	#1000	$51.00	Riker (Rauwiloid®)

Rauwolfia Serpentina, N.F. (whole root)

50 mgm tablet	2.40	Allen
	1.80	Am. Quinine
	2.10	Carroll
	1.70	Columbia Med.
	2.40	Horton & Converse
	2.40	Panray
	2.60	Penhurst
	2.10	Rondex
	27.00	Squibb (Raudixin®)
	2.44	Supreme
	3.00	West-ward

deserpidine

0.1 mgm tablet	#1000	$19.98	Abbott (Harmonyl®)

Rescinnamine, N.F.

0.25 mgm tablet		36.78*	Pfizer (Moderil®)

Syrosingopine, N.F.

1 mgm tablet		42.75	CIBA (Singoserp®)

At least one drug house markets reserpine in the form of a timed-disintegration capsule. These capsules contain the drug in many small granules designed to dissolve at varying times after being swallowed. Since reserpine has a slow and cumulative pharmacological action anyway, there is no advantage to such a dosage form.

0.25 mgm reserpine "Spansule"	#1000	$46.00†	Smith Kline & French (Eskaserp®)

To complicate matters, there are some much-prescribed tablets and capsules which contain both reserpine and a sedative. One such tablet is:

15 mgm butabarbital plus 0.1 mgm reserpine	#1000	$29.25	McNeil (Butiserpine®)

It is doubtful that butabarbital has any advantage over phenobarbital. In any event, butabarbital is available as a generic for as little as $1.75 per thousand 15 milligram tablets. One tenth milligram reserpine, as shown above, is available for approximately $1 per 1000 tablets. In view of this, the cost of Butiserpine® seems a little on the high side.

Some other tablets combining reserpine and a sedative:

* Actual listing $18.39/500
† Actual listing $2.30/50

0.25 mgm reserpine plus 7.5 mgm pyrrobutamine phosphate (an antihistamine with a sedative side effect)	#1000	$18.69	Lilly (Sandril® with Pyronil®)
0.25 mgm deserpidine plus 30 mgm pentobarbital		38.50	Abbott (Harmonyl-N®)

Obviously, it is far less costly to the patient (or to the taxpayer, if the patient is receiving free care from a municipal institution) to avoid the combinations. If a sedative is needed in addition to the reserpine, it takes only a moment more to write two prescriptions, one for reserpine tablets, 0.1 milligram, and another for phenobarbital, 15 or 30 milligrams.

THIAZIDES AND CONGENERS

Thiazides are diuretics which can be taken by mouth, instead of having to be injected as do most mercury-containing diuretics. They cause increased urine production and an increased excretion of salts in the urine. All diuretic drugs (including the mercurials) have a blood-pressure-lowering effect, and when they are given in conjunction with one or more other antihypertension agents, there is often a striking potentiation of the therapeutic effect (sometimes dangerously so). The most commonly employed drug regimen for treatment of high blood pressure is reserpine plus a thiazide. It is for this reason that the medical journals are glutted with advertisements for pharmaceuticals containing both agents in the same capsule or tablet. The use of such combinations is to be deplored. Not only are they unconscionably expensive, but in using them the physician loses independent dose control: he is stuck with a fixed ratio of doses which may not be the best for that particular patient. The combinations are widely used because of effective advertising and because the busy doctor need write only one prescription rather than two. The patient pays the price.

In choosing a thiazide for prescription, *the physician should remember that with respect to action the only major differences between them concern duration of action and that the best measurable criterion to use is price.* At present the least expensive in this family of drugs, all of which must still be bought by brand name, is Lakeside Laboratory's brand of trichlormethiazide, sold as Metahydrin®. Four milligrams is equieffective in respect to both diuretic and antihypertensive effects with 500 milligrams of chlorothiazide and 50 milligrams of hydrochlorothiazide.

TRICHLORMETHIAZIDE			
4 mgm tablet	#1000	$31.97	Lakeside (Metahydrin®)
		45.36	Schering (Naqua®)
Chlorothiazide, N.F.			
0.5 gm tablet (500 mgm)		52.73	Merck Sharp & Dohme (Diuril®)
Hydrochlorothiazide, U.S.P.			
0.05 gm tablet (50 mgm)		52.73	Merck Sharp & Dohme (Hydrodiuril®)
		57.00	CIBA (Esidrix®)
		57.00	Abbott (Oretic®)
bendroflumethiazide			
5 mgm tablet		50.00*	Bristol Labs (Benuron®)
		51.30	Squibb (Naturetin®)

* Actual listing $3.00/60

benzthiazide			
50 mgm tablet	#1000	$56.00*	A. H. Robins (Exna®) (Formerly NaClex®)
cyclothiazide			
2 mgm tablet		47.22	Lilly (Anhydron®)
hydroflumethiazide			
50 mgm tablet		60.00†	Bristol Labs (Saluron®)
methyclothiazide			
5 mgm tablet		57.00	Abbott (Enduron®)
polythiazide			
2 mgm tablet		48.45	Pfizer (Renese®)
chlorthalidone			
100 mgm tablet		59.40	Geigy (Hygroton®)
quinethazone			
50 mgm tablet		57.00‡	Lederle (Hydromox®)

There are many combinations of reserpine or a reserpine-like drug, but the doctor would be well advised to write individual prescriptions for reserpine and the least costly thiazide diuretic. This would constitute better therapeutic technique and would cost the patient less. Some of the presently popular combinations (in tablet form) and their cost follow.

* Actual listing $28.00/500
† Actual listing $3.00/50
‡ Actual listing $28.50/500

2 mgm cyclothiazide plus 0.25 mgm reserpine plus 500 mgm potassium chloride	#1000	$61.74	Lilly (Anhydron KR®)
5 mgm methyclothiazide plus 0.25 mgm deserpidine		81.50	Abbott (Enduronyl®)
5 mgm methyclothiazide plus 0.5 mgm deserpidine		94.00	Abbott (Enduronyl Forte®)
50 mgm benzthiazide plus 0.125 mgm reserpine		76.00*	A. H. Robins (Exna-R®)
500 mgm chlorothiazide plus 0.125 mgm reserpine		75.05	Merck Sharp & Dohme (Diupres-500®)
50 mgm chlorthalidone plus 0.25 mgm reserpine		54.00	Geigy (Regroton®)
50 mgm hydrochlorothiazide plus 0.125 mgm reserpine		75.05	Merck Sharp & Dohme (Hydropres-50®)
50 mgm quinethazone plus 0.125 mgm reserpine		75.04†	Lederle (Hydromox-R®)
4 mgm trichlormethiazide plus 0.1 mgm reserpine		50.75	Lakeside (Metatensin®)
		60.00‡	Schering (Naquival®)
50 mgm Rauwolfia serpentina whole root plus 4 mgm bendroflumethiazide plus 400 mgm potassium chloride		65.50	Squibb (Rautrax-N®)
2 mgm polythiazide plus 0.25 mgm reserpine		76.50§	Pfizer (Renese-R®)
"tablet 2"—50 mgm hydrochlorothiazide plus 0.1 mgm reserpine		71.29	CIBA (Serpasil-Esidrix® tablet #2)

* Actual listing $38.00/500
† Actual listing $37.52/500
‡ Actual listing $6.00/100
§ Actual listing $7.65/100

Some of these are seen to contain potassium chloride. The reason for this is that thiazide diuretics cause an increased loss of potassium in the urine along with sodium and water. If a patient is on a less than adequate diet, daily potassium intake could theoretically be (and sometimes actually is) less than urinary loss, and depletion of potassium can cause serious illness. It is a simple matter to prescribe two or three 300 milligram potassium chloride tablets if there is really any concern over adequacy of intake.* One thousand 300 milligram potassium chloride tablets can be bought for as little as $2.45 by the druggist. However, a daily glass or two of orange juice, a banana, or some figs usually suffice to supply supplemental potassium. At this point emphasis is again given to the fact that in the majority of patients mild or moderate hypertension can be satisfactorily controlled with reserpine plus a thiazide. For practical purposes there is little reason for the doctor to burden his mind with anything more than: reserpine tablets, 0.1 milligram, and trichlormethiazide (Lakeside), 4 milligrams.

Unfortunately (for it adds to the confusion), there are combinations of thiazides with sedatives. The following are in tablet form. (Separate prescriptions for phenobarbital plus the least expensive thiazide are equally effective and always less costly.)

25 mgm hydrochlorothiazide plus 30 mgm butabarbital	#500	$22.05	McNeil (Butizide®)
150 mgm metabumate plus 12.5 mgm hydrochlorothiazide	#100	5.00	Wallace (Caplaril®)
25 mgm hydrochlorothiazide plus 200 mgm meprobamate	#100	7.00	Merck Sharp & Dohme (Cyclex®)

There are even preparations with three components!

25 mgm hydrochlorothiazide plus 30 mgm butabarbital plus 0.1 mgm reserpine	#500	$27.00	McNeil (Butiserpazide-25®)

* Plain rather than enteric-coated tablets are preferred. The latter have been known rarely to cause serious inflammation of the small intestine.

The foregoing section is as illustrative as any other of the senseless proliferation of drugs nearly the same in all respects, each with its own name, and of overpriced combinations. Surely the situation as outlined above should be enough to convince anyone who has hitherto believed otherwise that it is easier as well as desirable to remember a very few generic names than a few score brand names.

THREE SOMETIMES USEFUL DRUGS

METHYLDOPA

An interesting and sometimes useful compound with a structure sufficiently similar to one of the important precursors of norepinephrine that the body's norepinephrine-synthesizing machinery is fooled into trying to convert it into norepinephrine. As a result, the sympathetic nerve endings (important in control of blood pressure) find themselves filled with a false transmitter rather than the normal transmitter, norepinephrine. Until very recently this was held to be the basis of methyldopa's ability to lower blood pressure, but now there is speculation among pharmacologists that its blood-pressure-lowering effect is due to an action on the brain. The drug is available from only one source at present, is expensive, is not without toxicity, but is sometimes very useful.

250 mgm tablet	#100	$6.00	Merck Sharp & Dohme (Aldomet®)

GUANETHIDINE SULFATE, U.S.P.

A powerful, effective drug for treating patients with severe high blood pressure which will not respond to reserpine, or reserpine plus a thiazide, or a thiazide plus methyldopa.

Guanethidine is like reserpine in that it causes depletion of the neuro-transmitter stores of sympathetic nerve fibers, but it probably has some additional action upon the sympathetic nerve endings (bretylium-like action) because it is more powerful by far than reserpine as a blood-pressure-lowering drug; so powerful, in fact, that unwanted side effects are common and patients require careful follow-up by a physician who has a good working knowledge of the physiology of the autonomic nervous system. While guanethidine administration will most commonly be initiated in the hospital, therapy may be continued in the non-hospitalized patient.

10 mgm tablet #1000 $63.90 CIBA (Ismelin®)

HYDRALAZINE HYDROCHLORIDE, N.F.

No one knows for certain even the *site* of action of this drug, not to mention its *mechanism* of action, but its effect is often to cause a fall in blood pressure. It makes the heart work harder, however, and this can sometimes be a disadvantage. When added to a regimen which already contains guanethidine, or guanethidine plus a thiazide, hydralazine may contribute key additional blood-pressure-lowering benefit. Some patients get fever and arthritis from hydralazine, and the drug may have to be discontinued.

10 mgm tablet #1000 $15.05 CIBA (Apresoline®)

An average daily dose is 3 or 4 tablets.

GANGLION-BLOCKING DRUGS

All the drugs in this group block both the sympathetic and parasympathetic divisions of the autonomic nervous system. Although they are capable of causing a good fall in blood pressure, especially when given in conjunction with one or more of the drugs mentioned earlier, unwanted side effects are usually encountered. Their administration is restricted to those few patients with the most severe forms of high blood pressure and should be carried out, initially at least, under supervision of someone experienced with their pharmacology. There are many contraindications to their use. Two of the more useful of these drugs are:

MECAMYLAMINE HYDROCHLORIDE, U.S.P.

2.5 mgm tablet	#100	$2.40	Merck Sharp & Dohme (Inversine®)

chlorisondamine chloride

25 mgm tablet		2.80	CIBA (Ecolid®)

Ganglion-blocking agents, guanethidine, hydralazine, and methyldopa will not have to be called upon for use as often as reserpine and thiazides. For the physician, the availability of agents is simple and clear; he need know only these six categories, and because most patients will respond either to reserpine and/or a thiazide, he need carry in his head only two generic names: reserpine and trichlormethiazide (Lakeside).

XII. Drugs for Heart Disease (Exclusive of Those Used to Treat High Blood Pressure)

DIGITALIS GLYCOSIDES

DIGITALIS, U.S.P. (DIGITALIS LEAF)

(Also officially "Powdered Digitalis.")

This is the dried leaves of the *Digitalis purpurea* plant pressed into tablets. It is one of the oldest and most reliable drugs known. Originally used as a folk remedy in Shropshire, England, for patients with "dropsy" (which we now call "heart failure"), it was carefully studied by the English physician William Withering, who in 1785 described its remarkable beneficial effects on the dropsical patient. Digitalis acts by increasing the force and efficiency of heart-muscle contraction, but exactly how it does this is unknown.

0.1 gm tablet	#1000	$ 1.36	Am. Quinine
		1.70	Carroll
		2.00	Corvit
		18.40*	Davies, Rose-Hoyt (Pil-Digis®)‡
		2.25	Horton & Converse
		1.90	Kasar
		2.20	Lannett
		2.50	Lederle
		6.72†	Lilly
		8.70†	Massengill
		17.55†	McNeil
		2.50	Merck Sharp & Dohme
		7.98	Parke, Davis (Digifortis®)
		2.35	Penhurst
		3.25	Stanlabs
		2.40	West-ward

DIGITOXIN, U.S.P.

The purified major active ingredient in digitalis leaf.

0.1 mgm tablet	#1000	$5.04	Abbott
		2.80	Allen Pharm.
		1.52	Am. Quinine
		1.95	Carroll
		1.45	Columbia Med.
		2.40	Corvit
		2.45	Daniels
		2.50	Horton & Converse
		1.90	Kasar
		2.20	Lannett
		6.06§	Lilly (Crystodigin®)
		5.04	Parke, Davis
		2.45	Penhurst

* Actual listing $1.84/100
† Capsules, not tablets
‡ Pills, not tablets
§ Actual listing $3.03/500

		2.25	Pennex
		2.25	Rondex
		5.04	Squibb
		2.90	Stayner
		2.79	Supreme
		3.25	Towne, Paulsen
		5.16*	Upjohn
		1.50	Vita-Fore
		2.89	Vitarine
		2.80	West-ward

DIGOXIN, U.S.P.

A purified active principle of the leaves of the plant *Digitalis lanata*. The beneficial effect on the failing heart is the same as that of digitalis leaf (whose major active principle is digitoxin). However, digoxin is distinctly different in that it is much more rapidly eliminated by the body than digitoxin. After administration of a single dose half of the digoxin in the body is eliminated in two days, whereas it takes nine days to get rid of half of a single dose of digitoxin. This property of digoxin makes it specially useful in many clinical situations.

0.25 mgm tablet	#1000	$5.40	Allen Pharm.
		4.48	Am. Quinine
		8.00	Burroughs Wellcome (Lanoxin®)
		4.75	Carroll
		4.10	Columbia Med.
		7.25	Corvit
		5.45	Daniels
		7.20	Horton & Converse
		5.80	Lannett
		5.95	Penhurst
		5.25	Rondex
		8.00	Sandoz
		5.50	Supreme

*Actual listing $2.58/500

		7.50	Towne, Paulsen
		3.75	Vita-Fore
		6.12	Vitarine
		5.50	West-ward

BLOOD VESSEL DILATORS

NITROGLYCERIN, U.S.P. (GLYCERYL TRINITRATE)

The essential first-choice agent for alleviation of angina pectoris, nitroglycerin was introduced more than one hundred years ago. There is still question as to how it works, but there is no doubt of its efficacy. It must be dissolved under the tongue for adequate absorption. Its cost is slight.

0.6 mgm tablet	#1000	$1.00	Lannett
(.01 gr)		2.10	Lilly
		2.10	Parke, Davis
		1.65	Penhurst

There are some curious entities sold for treatment of angina pectoris. One small company which specializes in combinations sold by brand name sells a capsule containing 2.5 milligrams of nitroglycerin plus a small dose of nicotinic acid, 35 milligrams. The nitroglycerin part is unreliable since absorption from the stomach and intestine is variable, unpredictable, and minimal. The nicotinic acid part is barely enough to provide a transient flushing of the skin. Value of the ingredients is less than $5 per 1000 doses. The cost to the druggist for the tablet is $42 per 1000!

pentaerythritol tetranitrate

This is quite an old chemical, available to the druggist from a large number of sources for as little as $2 to $4 per thousand 10 milligram doses. It was introduced initially as a nitroglycerine-like drug with a less intense but more sustained action for treatment of angina pectoris, but enthusiasm for the substance waned and for a decade or more it was little used. However, prescription of pentaerythritol has experienced a resurgence in recent years, stimulated largely by an intensive promotional campaign. There is much honest difference of opinion among doctors as to its value, and there are theoretical reasons for thinking that it could be harmful. Some believe it is nothing more than a placebo; others, that it is an effective vasodilator for the patient taking the first few doses only, and that with continued use it becomes ineffective ("tolerance"). One reason for the divergence of opinion is that angina pectoris is a symptom whose severity is well known to wax and wane spontaneously and even to benefit or worsen from psychological stimuli. In any event, because tolerance can develop rapidly to the effects of this and related compounds, if the drug is used at all, dosage should be kept at a minimum and slow-release dosage forms avoided.

10 mgm tablet	#1000	$ 3.60	Allen Pharm.
		2.70	Am. Quinine
		19.00	Amfre-Grant (Neo-Corovas®)
		2.40	Carroll
		1.85	Columbia Med.
		2.70	Corvit
		5.25	Daniels
		4.00	Lannett
		3.95	Penhurst
		2.50	Pennex
		3.60	Rondex
		1.50	Vita-Fore
		20.00*	Warner-Chilcott (Peritrate®)
		6.05	West-ward

DRUGS FOR CERTAIN ABNORMAL HEART RHYTHMS

QUINIDINE SULFATE, U.S.P.

Many instances of irregular heartbeat are helped by quinidine, one of the most useful of known drugs. It is a natural

* Actual listing $10.00/500

constituent in the bark of the cinchona tree, along with quinine, whose structure is a mirror image (stereoisomer) of quinidine. In spite of this seemingly small difference, quinidine has more effect on heart function than quinine. A Dutch sea captain is credited with first having drawn attention to the usefulness of quinine as a heart drug; he was subject to spontaneous paroxysms of irregular, rapid heartbeat. He was a frequent visitor to Dutch East Indian ports where malaria was rampant and where cinchona bark was universally self-administered by the population for fever from whatever cause. In fact, the popularity of cinchona bark was such that it came to be used indiscriminately for a wide variety of ills (much like aspirin today). The sea captain discovered that his irregular heartbeat was favorably affected by cinchona and so informed his European doctor, one Wenkebach, who in 1914 described the phenomenon in the medical literature. The greater efficacy of quinidine over quinine as a drug for heart disease was not discovered until a few years later.

Until very recently quinidine—and quinine, for that matter—were inexpensive. For many years the United States government held a vast stockpile of both substances to assure that in case of another world war our needs could be met, and the immensity of the stockpile had a beneficial economic effect: the single foreign cartel which controls the sources of these drugs was motivated to keep the price down lest our government be tempted to dump some of its reserve on the domestic market. Then, inexplicably, our State Department sold the greater part of it to the foreign cartel. This sale took place over the objections of the Justice Department, which pointed out that where there is monopoly, price is not determined by free competition, and as was predicted, the cost of the cinchona drugs was suddenly pegged at an artificially high level. The price is "administered," as the late Senator Kefauver would have said—set to bring in every penny the traffic will bear.

Many pharmaceutical distributors now limit the amount of

quinidine which they will sell to retailers, and the price is a function of availability. At present, fall 1966, pharmacists must pay about $60 per thousand 0.2 gram tablets. There is no sense in listing sources and prices because the situation is too unpredictable.

Fortunately, procainamide, which is manufactured domestically, can be substituted in most cases for quinidine.

PROCAINAMIDE HYDROCHLORIDE, U.S.P.

250 mgm capsule	#1000	$16.00	Interstate Drug Exchange (This is material manufactured by Nysco Labs, Inc.)
250 mgm capsule		27.00	Squibb (Pronestyl®)

THIAZIDES AND CONGENERS (See Section XI, pages 127–32)

XIII. Drugs for Gastrointestinal Disorders, Including Peptic Ulcer

BELLADONNA TINCTURE, U.S.P.

In order to make this very old-fashioned but wonderfully effective drug, 10 grams of the powdered leaves of the deadly nightshade plant are extracted into 100 milliliters (about 3 ounces) of a water-alcohol mixture. Ten grams of the powder costs the pharmaceutical manufacturer or druggist about 3.6 cents. Therefore, this drug is very inexpensive; this is fortunate, for it is the drug of choice to reduce hydrochloric acid secretion in the stomach and to cause considerable muscular relaxation within the gastrointestinal tract. Another big advantage is that it lends itself to flexibility of dosage. To find the proper dose for any given person is easy; the patient simply increases the number of drops he takes from day to day until he develops either a dry mouth or trouble focusing the eyes on near objects. One or two drops less than the maximum tolerated dose is the one best suited to the patient; it produces a good effect on the gastrointestinal tract with a minimum of side effects. Belladonna's disadvantages are minor: because it is a partially alcoholic solution, the bottle must be kept capped lest the vehicle evaporate and cause the active substance (atropine) to increase in concentration. Also, a small dropper bottle may be inconvenient to carry on the person.

The pharmacist can buy 450 cc belladonna tincture for less than $2.

Other belladonna-like drugs frequently prescribed are:

Methantheline Bromide, N.F.

50 mgm tablets	#500	$21.00	Searle (Banthine®)

Propantheline Bromide, U.S.P.

15 mgm tablets	#1000	36.00	Searle (Pro-Banthine®)

These are powerful substances whose net pharmacological effect is identical with that of belladonna tincture. However, since they act to block transmission of nerve impulses at two sites rather than one, in overdose they may cause a wider range of undesirable side effects. Aside from costliness, their major disadvantage is in their dosage form; as tablets they do not lend themselves to the nice adjustment of dose which is such a desirable feature of belladonna tincture. There is no advantage of propantheline over methantheline, or vice versa. The former is more potent, which is another way of saying that 15 milligrams is equal in effect to 50 milligrams of methantheline. This is of no advantage to the patient.

Methantheline is also sold in a tablet which combines 50 milligrams with 15 milligrams phenobarbital. The cost to the druggist is $4.80 per 100 tablets ($48 per 1000). This amounts to the druggist paying $6 per 1000 doses of phenobarbital which he is able to purchase alone for 75 cents or less. Similarly, propantheline may be obtained in a tablet which combines 15 milligrams with 15 milligrams phenobarbital at $39.60 per 1000 tablets, druggists' price. Aside from the cost issue, prescribing combinations of drugs in the same tablet or capsule is generally neither good practice nor necessary.

Dioctyl Sodium Sulfosuccinate, N.F.

Also known as dioctyl sodium succinate, this detergent material has a useful softening action on stools, allowing water and fats to permeate them. For the bedridden or elderly in whom constipation is a serious problem due to hard, dry, impacted fecal material, the drug can be helpful. Known almost exclusively to doctors and public alike by an expensive brand name, the substance is readily available at reasonable price from many sources.

100 mgm tablet or capsule #1000	$ 7.80	Am. Quinine
	8.50*	Carroll
	6.00	Corvit
	8.50	Daniels
	8.00	Lannett
	45.79	Mead Johnson (Colace®)
	7.50	Rondex
	9.00	Stayner
	9.00	Towne, Paulsen
	5.95	Vita-Fore
	10.15	West-ward

MAGNESIUM AND ALUMINUM HYDROXIDE SUSPENSION

This mixture, suspended in a flavored vehicle, is now the most widely used antacid and is practically always prescribed by brand name. The presence of the magnesium causes the bowels to be a little loose. Many other antacid preparations cause constipation.

* Actual listing $.85/100

15 oz bottle	$ .46	Carroll
12 " "	.48	Columbia Med.
12 " "	.60	Penhurst
12 " "	.45	Pennex
12 " "	.50	Rondex
12 " "	1.05	Rorer (Maalox®)
12 " "	.55	Vita-Fore
12 " "	.55	Vitarine

PAREGORIC, U.S.P. (CAMPHORATED TINCTURE OF OPIUM)

Far and away the most effective antidiarrheal agent for use in ambulatory patients. The fact that it is camphorated discourages excessive oral intake. One gallon of paregoric costs the druggist as little as $6, so the one-ounce bottle which he may sell over the counter without a prescription in many states has a wholesale value of about 5 cents. Compare this with the cost of the following:

2.5 mgm tablet, diphenoxylate hydrochloride plus 0.025 mgm atropine sulfate	#100	$6.00	Searle (Lomotil®)

XIV. Adrenal Steroids

ORAL PREPARATIONS

It is common knowledge that with few exceptions patients who require treatment with oral corticosteroids can be taken care of satisfactorily with prednisone. Unless therapy is to be with high dosage for a long period, fluid retention is rarely a serious side effect. The point is that it is rarely necessary to prescribe those steroids alleged to have fewer salt-retaining properties except in exceptional instances. The cost difference between prednisone and the others is very great.

PREDNISONE, U.S.P.

5 mgm tablet	#1000	$ 8.95	Allen Pharm.
		8.75	Carroll
		7.95	Columbia Med.
		8.95	Daniels
		10.98	Horton & Converse
		9.40	Lannett
		20.90*	Merck Sharp & Dohme (Deltra®)
		7.50	Panray
		169.98	Parke, Davis (Paracort®)
		8.50	Penhurst
		9.45	Pennex
		8.95	Rondex
		170.00	Schering (Meticorten®)
		15.00	Stayner
		8.95	Supreme
		14.35	Towne, Paulsen
		20.94	Upjohn (Deltasone®)
		20.00	U.S. Vitamin
		10.16	Vitarine
		11.95	West-ward

A host of adrenal cortex steroids are available, including such early ones as cortisone and hydrocortisone. The use of these two as oral medications has largely been supplanted by prednisone, for prednisone causes significantly less salt and water retention. In recent years a growing list of synthetic steroids has appeared to the tune of various advertising claims, but the practicing physician can handle nearly all clinical situations requiring oral adrenal steroid treatment with prednisone, now an official drug of the *United States Pharmacopeia*.

Introduced at about the same time as prednisone was prednisolone, very similar in structure, potency, and activity. The two are interchangeable. Prednisolone, available as a generic, is

* Actual listing $10.45/500

marketed by more than eighty companies (prices are practically the same as those of prednisone). However, prednisolone too is sold under brand name at high prices.

Prednisolone, U.S.P.

5 mgm tablet	#1000	$24.50*	Merck Sharp & Dohme (Hydeltra®)
		169.98	Parke, Davis (Paracortol®)
		17.00	Pfizer (Sterane®)
		170.00	Schering (Meticortelone®)
		23.94	Upjohn (Delta-Cortef®)

Synthetic steroids newer than prednisone and prednisolone have been marketed, all of high potency and even less likely to cause salt retention than prednisone and prednisolone. However, salt and water retention due to prednisone is rarely troublesome clinically and can usually be controlled easily by limiting salt intake and by judicious prescription of diuretic drugs. Potency is of no practical importance: what should the patient care if the tablet he swallows contains 5 or 0.5 milligrams of active drug?

Methylprednisolone, N.F.

4 mgm tablet	#1000	$145.35	Upjohn (Medrol®)

Dexamethasone Sodium Phosphate, N.F.

0.75 mgm tablet		153.92†	CIBA (Gammacorten®)
		137.70	Merck Sharp & Dohme (Decadron®)
		80.00‡	Organon (Hexadrol®)
		153.90§	Schering (Deronil®)
		58.00	U.S. Vitamin (Dexameth®)

* Actual listing $2.45/100
† Actual listing $38.48/250
‡ Actual listing $8.00/100
§ Actual listing $76.95/500

Dexamethasone and other even more potent chemicals *are* of great importance as *research* tools.

triamcinolone

Triamcinolone is a steroid which causes even less salt retention than either methylprednisolone or dexamethasone. Its anti-inflammation properties are quite satisfactory. Its disadvantage is that it is not only capable of causing all the toxic effects of prednisone, prednisolone, methylprednisolone, and dexamethasone, but is also likely to cause flushing of the face, muscle cramps, sweating, mental depression, and a peculiar weakness of pelvic, trunk, and shoulder muscles.

4 mgm tablets	#1000	$144.50	Lederle (Aristocort®)
		144.50	Squibb (Kenacort®)

TOPICAL PREPARATIONS

In office practice, one of the most useful preparations available for treatment of many skin disorders is ointment or washable cream containing steroid. A large number of these are marketed by brand name, usually in collapsible tubes, and they are all very high-priced. The least costly way to obtain a substantial amount is to have a pharmacist make it up. He simply disperses hydrocortisone (which has the same actions as other steroids) in a water-soluble base (cream) or petrolatum (ointment). Since hydrocortisone powder costs the druggist approximately $15 for 10 grams, the amount required to make up 3 ounces of cream or ointment of 1% strength is worth $1.50 wholesale cost. He may fairly charge $2.50 for it. Three ounces of petrolatum costs the druggist less than 10 cents and a similar amount of Burroughs Wellcome's greaseless ointment ("Neobase") about 35 cents. Thus, including a charge for compounding, the druggist ought to be able to sell about 100 grams (3 ounces) of cream or ointment for about \$3.50. Steroid cream or ointment bought by well-advertised brand name is two to three times as costly.

Some available preparations with hydrocortisone:

HYDROCORTISONE OINTMENT, U.S.P. (or cream) (1%)

20 gm tube	\$ 1.20 (\$12.75/doz)	Columbia Med.
15 " "	2.71	Dome Chemicals (Cort-Dome® Creme)
450 " (1 lb)	14.00 (\$2.00/oz)	Horton & Converse
450 " "	11.50 (\$1.50/oz)	Penhurst
20 gm tube	1.00	Pennex
15 " "	1.10	Pfizer (Cortril® Topical Ointment)
20 " "	1.65	Rondex
20 " "	1.75	Stanlabs
20 " "	1.56 (\$18.75/doz)	Supreme
20 " "	2.85	Upjohn (Cortef Ointment®)
20 " "	1.60	West-ward

Some other brand-name preparations with steroids for topical use:

Aristocort® Topical Cream (0.1% triamcinolone)	15 gm tube	\$1.78	Lederle
Aristocort® Topical Ointment (0.1% triamcinolone)	" "	1.78	Lederle
Celestone® Cream (0.2% betamethasone)	" "	2.22	Schering
Cordran® Cream (.05% flurandrenolone)	" "	1.89	Lilly
Decadron® Topical Cream (0.1% Dexamethasone Sodium Phosphate, U.S.P.)	" "	1.51	Merck Sharp & Dohme
Kenalog® Cream (0.1% triamcinolone)	" "	1.87	Squibb

Kenalog® Ointment (0.1% triamcinolone)	15 gm tube	1.87	Squibb
Kenalog® Cream or Ointment (0.025% triamcinolone)	60 " "	2.63	Squibb
Meti-Derm® Cream (0.5% Prednisolone Sodium Phosphate, U.S.P.)	10 " "	1.90	Schering
Oxylone® Cream (.025% fluorometholone)	7.5 " "	0.98	Upjohn
Synalar® Cream or Ointment (.025% fluocinolone)	15 " "	1.90	Syntex
Synalar® Cream (0.01% fluocinolone)	45 " "	2.90	Syntex

XV. Oral Contraceptives and Female Hormones

ORAL CONTRACEPTIVES

A natural situation in which it is impossible for man to impregnate woman is where the woman is already pregnant. This is because the abundant production in pregnancy of one of the female hormones, progesterone, inhibits the release of new eggs (ovulation) and has myriad other effects as well. Deliberate "molecule manipulating" on the part of chemists has resulted in a variety of compounds (progestogens) whose ability to inhibit ovulation remains intact while many other effects are minimized; it was fortunate that the effect of progesterone on ovulation was able to be dissociated from its other actions. By combining a progestogen with estrogen, another female hormone, a state reminiscent of pregnancy (pseudopregnancy) is induced. This explains the transient morning nausea or vomiting, painful swelling of the breasts, and occasional pigmentation of the face which can accompany the taking of these drugs.

The *Handbook* simply lists identity, source, and price with no implication whatsoever as to relative or absolute efficacy or safety, preferring to delay in deciding whether these are to be considered basic drugs.

Ethinyl Estradiol, U.S.P. plus dimethisterone with Ethinyl Estradiol	21 tablets	$1.35	Mead Johnson (Oracon®)
medroxyprogesterone with Ethinyl Estradiol	6 packs, 20 tablets each	6.60	Upjohn (Provest®)
mestranol plus chlormadinone with mestranol	6 packs, 20 tablets each	8.10	Lilly (C-Quens®)
2 mgm norethindrone with 0.1 mgm mestranol	5 packs, 20 tablets each	6.60	Syntex (Norinyl®)
" "	6 packs, 20 tablets each	8.10	Ortho (Ortho-Novum®)
norethindrone with Ethinyl Estradiol	100 tablets	6.54	Parke, Davis (Norlestrin®)
2.5 mgm norethynodrel with 0.1 mgm mestranol	6 packs, 20 tablets each	8.10	Searle (Enovid-E®)

FEMALE HORMONES (NO CONTRACEPTIVE ACTION)

DIETHYLSTILBESTROL, U.S.P.

The discovery that this synthetic chemical, easy and cheap to make, will mimic all of the estrogenic effects of natural female hormones, can be taken by mouth, and does not have to be injected in order to be effective is one of pharmacology's most fascinating chapters. Physicians and others interested in this intriguing story are referred to Sir Charles Dodds's recent review in *The Scientific Basis of Medicine* (Athlone Press, University of London, 1965). The laborious efforts of a group of dedicated laboratory scientists interested in structure-activity relationships among female hormones attracted little attention until 1938, when they demonstrated the properties of diethylstilbestrol, a substance which until then had never been synthesized by organic chemists. Diethylstilbestrol is now one of medicine's basic drugs.

1 mgm tablet, enteric coated	#1000	$2.40	Allen Pharm.
		1.60	Carroll
		1.50	Columbia Med.
		2.25	Daniels
		2.00	Horton & Converse
		2.10	Lannett
		6.30	Lilly
		2.25	Penhurst
		3.05	Pennex
		1.60	Rondex
		8.00*	Squibb (Stilbetin®)
		2.60	Stayner
		4.00	Towne, Paulsen
		8.28	Upjohn
		1.95	Vita-Fore
		2.55	West-ward

conjugated estrogenic derivatives

It is presently fashionable to prescribe this drug for various conditions—most commonly for menopausal symptoms. Whether it has any advantage over diethystilbestrol is not known, but it is certainly more expensive. The material is isolated from the urine of female horses.

0.625 mgm tablet	#1000	$35.40	Ayerst Labs (Premarin®)
		16.00	Corvit
		17.00	Daniels

* Actual listing $.80/100

XVI. Vitamins

There is probably more indiscriminate prescribing and self-dosing with vitamin preparations than with any other drug or combination of drugs available in pharmacies today. The immense lucrativeness of the market is evidenced by the inclusion in the 1966 *Physicians' Desk Reference* alone of more than three hundred different dosage forms with various combinations of vitamins, and combinations of vitamins with minerals. Without entering into a discussion of the pros and cons of whether supplemental intake of vitamins is desirable for the average North American, doctors and their patients should be aware that there is only one official multivitamin preparation in the *United States Pharmacopeia*. Called Decavitamin Capsules or Decavitamin Tablets (they have the identical constituents), each dose contains:

Vitamin A 4000 units
Vitamin D 400 units
Vitamin C 75 milligrams
Vitamin B complex
- thiamine (B_1) 1.0 milligram
- riboflavin (B_2) 1.2 milligrams
- nicotinamide (niacinamide) 10 milligrams
- folic acid 0.25 milligram (250 micrograms)
- pyridoxine (B_6) 2.0 milligrams
- calcium pantothenate 5 milligrams
- cyanocobalamin (B_{12}) 2 micrograms

No "therapeutic" concentrate, inordinately rich in multivitamins, is any longer official in the *U.S.P.* Each of the components of a Decavitamin Capsule or Tablet is present in an amount which approximates the Recommended Daily Dietary Allowance of the National Academy of Sciences–National Research Council. However, among experts, there is serious question even with respect to this official mixture as to the advisability of including folic acid in such a large dose, but a discussion of this point is beyond the scope of the *Handbook*.

The *United States Pharmacopeia* has chosen to design a multiple-vitamin preparation because it is a fact that persons who for any reason are truly vitamin-deficient rarely lack only one. Pernicious anemia, which is due to vitamin B_{12} deficiency, may be cited as an exception, but here the diet contains adequate B_{12}; the patient is simply unable to absorb it from the intestine. (The amount of B_{12} in Decavitamins is not enough to have a favorable effect in a patient with pernicious anemia.)

Aside from the question of folic acid's inclusion, there is little or no threat to health posed by excessive intake of the remainder of the B complex of vitamins and vitamin C because all are water-soluble and when the body is saturated with any one, the ingested excess goes out in the urine. Health may not suffer, but money has been spent unnecessarily. On the other hand, the amounts of the fat-soluble vitamins A and D which are taken either in supplements to the diet or in the diet itself are of critical importance, for the body has no way to get rid of excess and literally poisonous quantities can accumulate. Children taking upward of 50,000 units of vitamin A daily for six months or more have developed serious illness. Vitamin D intoxication is more common and is a very serious disease, marked among other things by deposition of insoluble calcium salts in the kidneys. It has been reliably stated that continued ingestion of 150,000 units or more of vitamin D daily may result in poisoning. A glance at the contents of an official Decavitamin Capsule or Tablet will reassure the patient and doctor that daily ingestion of one is safe for adults. Children and infants are special cases; parents are advised to follow closely and not exceed the instructions of the family doctor or pediatrician.

The addition of minerals to preparations containing multiple vitamins deserves comment if only to be deplored. Inclusion of iron in therapeutic amounts makes a "shotgun" preparation, one which discourages careful diagnosis, leads to unnecessary expense, and prevents individual adjustment of vitamin dosages on one hand and of iron dosages on the other. For inclusion of such trace metals as zinc, copper, manganese, molybdenum, and cobalt in vitamin or iron preparations intended for human consumption, there is no justification. This is a "gimmick" which simply adds to the price.

The confusion which meets the busy doctor who wishes to choose a vitamin preparation for prescription defies description. In short, a careful search of all of the indexes in the *Physicians' Desk Reference* reveals nothing which suggests to the doctor that there is an official *U.S.P.* preparation containing multiple vitamins.

DECAVITAMIN CAPSULES, U.S.P. and
DECAVITAMIN TABLETS, U.S.P.

#1000	$4.80	Am. Quinine
	7.50	Consolidated Midland
	6.00	Lannett
	8.50	Merrell
	4.50	Panray
	8.50	Penhurst

XVII. Iron

Listed below are three simple preparations of iron, one of which will suffice to treat almost any person with iron-deficiency anemia who is able to swallow medication and does not suffer at the same time from certain abnormalities of the gastrointestinal tract (for such rare individuals there is a preparation of injectable iron). Of the three, *ferrous sulfate is the agent of choice because it is the least expensive.* Salts other than the sulfate have been introduced because of the widely held belief that many persons develop an upset stomach or diarrhea or constipation from ferrous sulfate. Actually, intolerance simply depends on *how much* iron is taken by mouth and is independent of the form in which it is administered. The way to avoid most trouble is to take the ferrous sulfate tablet immediately after a meal, starting with one tablet per day and slowly increasing to three per day after a week or two. The patient should know that his stool will turn black, which is no cause for alarm but could in rare instances make him overlook gastrointestinal bleeding, also a cause of black stools.

Warning: Iron preparations must absolutely be kept out of the reach of children. Most tablets are an attractive green or red color, often sugar- or even chocolate-coated; children mistake them for candy. Fatal poisoning can occur in infants and small children who swallow upward of half a dozen ordinary therapeutic iron tablets! Bottles should carry a warning label.

One of the most shameful examples of the extent to which detail men, Madison Avenue promoters, and the *PDR* have succeeded in confusing practicing doctors is in the way they have influenced prescription of iron preparations. They promote medications containing substances in addition to iron which are alleged to have advantages over iron alone, but these allegations have no convincing foundation. In the 1966 *PDR*, under fumarate, gluconate, and sulfate salts of ferrous iron, is listed a total of 114 different brand names. Of the 51 which contain ferrous fumarate, only 5 contain ferrous fumarate alone; only 1 of the 21 gluconate preparations is not a mixture; and only 4 of 42 sulfate preparations are marketed without the addition of an "adjuvant." Additives include ascorbic acid, folic acid, concentrates of liver and stomach, vitamin B_{12}, manganese, zinc, magnesium, copper, cobalt, inositol, choline, polysaccharide, and all the common vitamins. In some cases one wonders seriously how so much material can fit into a capsule or tablet small enough to swallow. The cost to the druggist of seven of the better known combinations (not necessarily the most expensive ones, either!) was found to range from $52 down to $22 per 1000 doses. An eighth, a well-advertised preparation which contains only one added ingredient, goes for $9. Ferrous sulfate and other ferrous salts are far too efficacious when given by themselves in the treatment of simple iron-deficiency anemia to warrant the costly addition of supplements.

The *Handbook* emphasizes that the only indication for iron therapy is iron deficiency; the indiscriminate taking of iron is not to be condoned, since there is a possibility that disease may be caused by excessive deposition of iron in certain organs. Finally, iron deficiency, while occasionally caused by inadequate diet, is most often a manifestation of excessive blood loss which in males and in females after the child-bearing age is reason for careful search on the part of the doctor for a bleeding lesion. Correction of the anemia with iron tablets should not be allowed to obscure this serious consideration.

FERROUS SULFATE, U.S.P.

0.3 gm tablet (5 gr) #1000	$ 2.00	Allen Pharm.
	1.32	Am. Quinine
	1.75	Carroll
	1.75	Columbia Med.
	2.00	Corvit
	1.95	Daniels
	3.75	Horton & Converse
	2.00	Lannett
	5.04	Lilly (Enseals—enteric-coated)
	3.30	Lilly (Tablets)
	5.04	Parke, Davis
	1.75	Penhurst
	2.05	Pennex
	1.85	Rondex
	9.00	Smith Kline & French (Feosol®)*
	3.25	Stanlabs
	1.95	Supreme

* 0.2 gm dried ferrous sulfate

	2.75	Towne, Paulsen
	3.30	Upjohn
	1.75	Vita-Fore
	2.10	Vitarine
	2.60	West-ward

Ferrous Fumarate, U.S.P.

0.3 gm tablet (5 gr)	#1000	$ 6.75	Corvit
		18.00*	Lakeside (Ircon®)
		5.50	Penhurst
		8.75	Towne, Paulsen
		5.35	West-ward

Ferrous Gluconate, N.F.

0.3 gm tablet (5 gr)	3.25	Carroll
	3.50	Corvit
	3.50	Daniels
	3.75	Horton & Converse
	2.90	Lannett
	9.15	Lilly
	2.95	Penhurst
	4.55	Stanlabs
	2.95	Vita-Fore
	4.35	West-ward

XVIII. Blood-Sugar-Lowering Drugs

INSULIN INJECTION, U.S.P.

The backbone of diabetes therapy. The history of insulin's discovery goes back to 1889 when two German investigators, Von Mering and Minkowski, studying digestive function in dogs, surgically removed the pancreas of several. Flies were attracted in larger numbers to the cages of these animals than to those of unoperated ones, and this was found to be due to the presence of large amounts of sugar in their urine. This was the first re-

* 0.2 gm tablet

corded intimation that the pancreas might have anything to do with "sugar diabetes," at that time a fatal disease in young persons. After unsuccessful attempts on the part of many researchers, Drs. Banting and Best at the University of Toronto succeeded in isolating from fresh pancreatic tissue a principle called "insulin," which on injection into a dying diabetic adolescent caused dramatic improvement. Subsequently isolated in pure form, insulin's complicated protein structure has in recent years been unraveled (1960), and only three years ago (1964) the hormone was actually synthesized. However, commercial insulin must still be extracted from slaughterhouse animal tissue, which makes it expensive, though no more so than the oral blood-sugar-lowering agents whose price was artificially set to be approximately the same as insulin's. Insulin is the agent of choice in every respect except convenience of administration, for it must be injected either by the patient himself or by someone else.

10 cc Regular Insulin U 80 (i.e. 80 units/cc)	$1.65	Squibb	
10 cc Globin Insulin U 80	1.89	"	
10 cc NPH Insulin U 80	1.89	"	
10 cc Protamine Zinc Insulin U 80	1.89	"	
10 cc Regular Insulin U 80	1.65	Lilly	(Iletin®)
10 cc Lente Insulin U 80	1.89	"	"
10 cc NPH Insulin U 80	1.89	"	"
10 cc Protamine Zinc Insulin U 80	1.89	"	"
10 cc Semi-lente Insulin U 80	1.89	"	"
10 cc Ultra-lente Insulin U 80	1.89	"	"

If you are a diabetic and your doctor wants you to take insulin, do what he says. Do not try to pressure him into prescribing tablets.

ORAL PREPARATIONS

Treatment of asymptomatic diabetes with these agents is investigational since neither the long-term benefits nor the hazards have been clearly defined. These drugs are indicated primarily for treatment of persons with onset of mild diabetes after age forty. They do not replace insulin in treatment of juvenile diabetes, "brittle diabetes," or diabetes when complicated by ketoacidosis, infection, or stress due to surgery or trauma. Three are sulfonamide derivatives, which allegedly act by causing the pancreas somehow to increase its output of insulin, and a fourth acts in an as yet unknown fashion.

Tolbutamide, U.S.P.

0.5 gm tablet	#500	$32.91	Upjohn (Orinase®)

Chlorpropamide, U.S.P.

0.25 gm tablet	#250	18.36	Pfizer (Diabinese®)

acetohexamide

0.25 gm tablet	#500	16.80	Lilly (Dymelor®)

In terms of cost alone, acetohexamide would appear to be the least expensive of the three agents in this group. On the other hand, it is still a less well known drug than the others, its date of introduction being 1964, as compared to 1957 for tolbutamide and 1958 for chlorpropamide. An interesting adverse effect of all three is the intolerance of alcohol which their users may experience.

phenformin

25 mgm tablet	#1000	$33.15	U.S. Vitamin (DBI®)

This material differs chemically from the three above. The mechanism of action is unknown, but it does not seem to act by causing more insulin release by the pancreas. The long-term value to human beings of merely lowering the blood-sugar level is not known.

Appendix A

Responsible Prospective Contractors for Drugs and Medical Supplies to the Defense Supply Agency of the United States

It has been made abundantly clear (see Table I) that the application of a brand name to a drug product is no guarantee of quality; reliability on the part of a pharmaceutical manufacturer is independent of corporate size and advertising budget. Yet it is only realistic to accept the likelihood that there are firms which are more reliable than others, and the doctor, pharmacist, and patient would like to be able to distinguish them, large or small. This appendix may help them to do so.

The taxpaying citizen has a right to know the identity of all pharmaceutical manufacturers who have met the inspection requirements of the Defense Supply Agency and are authorized to submit bids for contract from the government. A number are listed below, although the appearance of a firm's name does not necessarily imply over-all endorsement by the *Handbook*.

/ *Appendix A*

The companies listed in the following pages are qualified as "Responsible Prospective Contractors" with respect to drugs and medical supplies as defined in the Armed Services Procurement Regulations, Part 9, June 1965, Rev. 11. The list was supplied to me by a member of the staff of the United States Senate Select Committee on Small Business. It was compiled as of August 29, 1966. I hope that the list as supplied to me was complete, but cannot be responsible for inadvertent omissions from it. Obviously, there must be many more responsible corporations whose names are not listed here because they have never made application to the federal government for approval as bidders.

Most of the firms listed here are not mentioned in the *Handbook*. The primary purpose in publishing this list is to give emphasis to the fact that there are many manufacturers of drugs and medical supplies in addition to those whose names are household words.

Abbott Laboratories
Ace Scientific Supply Co., Inc.
Aceto Chemical Co., Inc.
Affiliated Distillers Brands Corp.
Air Products & Chemicals, Inc.
Alcon Laboratories, Inc.
Allen Metal Products, Inc.
Allen Pharmacal Co., Inc.
Allergan Pharmaceuticals, Inc.
Allied Chemical Corp.
Alrose Chemical Co.
Alta Pharmacal Corp.
Amend Drug & Chemical Co., Inc.
American Assoc. of Blood Banks
American Chemical Drug Co.
American Continental Laboratories
American Cryogenics, Inc.
American Cyanamid Co.
American Home Products Corp.
American Hospital Supply Corp.
American Lanolin Corp.
American Pharmaceutical Co.
Ames Company
Amole, Inc.
Amsco Laboratories
Anabolic Food Products, Inc.
Anderson Laboratories, Inc.
Anderson-Keith
Andor Laboratories, Inc.
Antigen Limited
Applied Biological Science Laboratory
Archer-Taylor Drug Co.
Arlin Chemical, Inc.

Armour & Co.
Armour Pharmaceutical Co.
Arnel Products Co.
Associated Chemists
Associated Laboratories, Inc.
Astra Pharmaceutical Products, Inc.
Avon Products, Inc.
Ayerst Laboratories
Baird & McGuire, Inc.
Baker, J. T. Chemical Co.
Baltimore Biological Laboratory
Banner Gelatin Products Corp.
Bard Pharmaceuticals, Inc.
Barium & Chemicals, Inc.
Barnes-Hind Pharmaceuticals
Barrows Chemical Co., Inc.
Barry Laboratories, Inc.
Barton Distilling Co.
Baxter, Don Inc.
Baxter Laboratories, Inc.
Bel-Art Products
Bellevue Labs, Inc.
Ben Venue Laboratories, Inc.
Berge, J & H Inc.
Berk, F. W. & Co.
Bethlehem Apparatus Co., Inc.
Biber Pharmacal Co., Inc.
Bio-Chem Products Co.
Biocraft Laboratories, Inc.
Bolar Pharmaceutical Co.
Bordon Chemical Co.
Bowman Bros. Drug Co.
Bowman Mell & Co.
Bowman-Braun Pharmaceuticals
Boyle & Co.
Breon Laboratories, Inc.
Brewer & Co., Inc.
Bristol Laboratories
Broemmel Pharmaceuticals
Brownlee, D. Co.
Bryant Laboratories, Inc.
Bryant Pharmaceutical Corp.
Buffalo Dental Mfg. Co.
Burroughs Wellcome & Co., Inc.
Burton Parsons & Co., Inc.
Butcher, L. H. Co.
Byars, David O.
C & M Pharmacal, Inc.
C P Chemical Solvents
Cambridge Chemical Products, Inc.
Can-Tite Rubber Corp.
Cargille, R. P. Laboratories, Inc.
Carlo Erba S P A
Carnegie Laboratories
Case Laboratories, Inc.
Central Pharmacal Co.
Certified Aspirin Corp.
Certified Blood Donor Service
Certified Laboratories, Inc.
Chase Chemical Co.
Chattanooga Medicine Co.
Chemical Compounding Corp.
Chemical Solvents, Inc.
Chemico Laboratories, Inc.
Chesebrough-Pond's, Inc.
Chicago Pharmacal Co.
Chicago Sanitary Products Co.
CIBA Pharmaceutical Co.
City Chemical Corp.
Colab Laboratories, Inc.
College of American Pathologists
Columbia Pharmaceutical Corp.
Comfort Manufacturing Co.
Community Blood Bank & Serum Service
Conal Pharmaceuticals, Inc.
Condit, P. N.

Consolidated Laboratories, Inc.
Consolidated Oxygen & Equipment Co., Inc.
Consolidated Products Corp.
Continental Chemical Co., Inc.
Continental Chemical Corp.
Cook-Waite Laboratories, Inc.
Cooper Chemical Co.
Cooper, Tinsley Laboratories, Inc.
Cord Laboratories, Inc.
Courtlandt Laboratories
Cowley Pharmaceuticals, Inc.
Crookes-Barnes Laboratories, Inc.
Crystal Soap & Chemical Co., Inc.
Custom Packaging, Inc.
Cutter Laboratories, Inc.
Dade Reagents, Inc.
Davies-Young Soap Co.
Davies Rose Hoyt
Day-Baldwin, Inc.
De Neve Pittsburg Shoes, Inc.
De Witt Chemical Co.
Delamar & Son, J. H., Inc.
Delmar Pharmacal Corp.
Delmar Scientific Laboratories
Delmond Pharmaceutical Corp.
Delta Biochemicals, Inc.
Delta Division
Denison Laboratories, Inc.
Denver Chemical Mfg. Co.
Derrick Soap Products
Derry Products, Inc.
Dewey Products Co.
Difco Laboratories, Inc.
Doak Pharmacal Co., Inc.
Dodge & Olcott, Inc.
Dome Chemicals, Inc.
Dorsey Laboratories
Dougherty's, J. A. Sons, Inc.
Dow Chemical Co.
Drug Package, Inc.
Drug Purchase, Inc.
Dumas-Wilson & Company
Dumont Pharmacal Co., Inc.
Durel Pharmaceutical Co., Inc.
Durst, S. F. & Co., Inc.
Duveen Soap Corp.
Eastman Kodak Distillation Products, Inc.
Eastern Laboratories, Inc.
Eastern Smelting & Refining Corp.
Eastern Wine Corp.
Eaton Laboratories
Eberbach & Son Co.
Economics Laboratory, Inc.
Edison, Thomas A. Industries
Edwards Councilor Co., Inc.
Elbon Laboratories, Inc.
Em, E. Z. Company, Inc.
Empire Laboratories Ltd.
Enjay Chemical Co.
Ethicon Inc.
Evans Chemetics, Inc.
FBA Pharmaceuticals, Inc.
Fine Organics, Inc.
Fisher Scientific Co.
Fleet Company, Inc., C. B.
Foregger Co., Inc.
Fort Dodge Laboratories, Inc.
Foster-Milburn Co.
Fougera & Co., E.
Four Penny Products, Inc.
Freibe RG & Son, E., Inc.
Fritzsche Bros., Inc.
Fromm & Sichel, Inc.
Fromm Laboratories, Inc.

G & W Laboratories, Inc.
Garfield & Co.
Gebauer Chemical Co.
Geigy Chemical Corp.
Giant Chemical Co.
Glenbrook Laboratories
Gold Leaf Pharmacal Co., Inc.
Goldsmith Bros. Division
Goldsmith, D. F. Chemical
Good, James, Inc.
Goodman Chemical N.Y. Corp.
Goodrich-Wright, Inc.
Gotham Pharmaceutical Co., Inc.
Grace, W. R. & Company
Grays Pharmacal Co.
Gryphon Laboratories Ltd.
Gyma Laboratories of America, Inc.
H & B Company
Haack Laboratories, Inc.
Halcarbon Laboratories, Inc.
Halperin, A. E. Co., Inc.
Halsey Drug Co., Inc.
Halsey X-ray Products, Inc.
Hance Bros. & White Co.
Harley Chemical, Inc.
Harriet Hubbard Ayer, Inc.
Harrisburg Steel Co.
Hart Laboratories, Inc.
Hartman-Leddon Co.
Harvey Laboratories, Inc.
Haver-Lockhart Laboratories
Hayward, George M.
Heico, Inc.
Hellige, Inc.
Hewitt Soap Co., Inc.
Hexagon Laboratories, Inc.
Heyden Newport Chemical Corp.
Hite, S. P. Co., Inc.
Hockwald Company
Holland-Rantos Co., Inc.
Honiberg Medical-Surgical Supply Co.
Hoppers Laboratories, Inc.
Horton & Converse
House of Hollywood
Hu-Friedy Inclinois
Hunt Manufacturing Co.
Huntington Labs, Inc.
Hutchinson, D. W. Co., Inc.
Hycel, Inc.
Hyland Laboratories
Hynson, Westcott & Dunning, Inc.
Imperial Wine Products
Industria Galenica Italiana
Inland Alkaloid Co.
International Bartering Corp.
International Chemical Corp.
Intra Products
Jamco Company
Jaymar Scientific Co.
Johnson Drug Co.
Johnson & Johnson
Josiassen Smelting Refining Co.
Kapco, Inc.
Kasar Laboratories
Keleket X-ray
Key Pharmaceuticals, Inc.
Kings Specialty Company
Kirk, C. F. Co.
Kirk, C. F. Laboratories, Inc.
Kirkman Laboratories, Inc.
Knoll Pharmaceutical Co.
Kohn, Herbert Co.
Konigslow, Otto Mfg. Co.
Koster Keunen, Inc.
Kremers-Urban Co.

Krylon, Inc.
Laboratories Atral S A R L
Laboratories Castillon SA
Laboratory Diagnostics Co.
Lafayette Pharmacal, Inc.
Lakeside Laboratories, Inc.
Lambert-Hudnut Manufacturing Labs, Inc.
Lamex, Inc.
Lannett Company, Inc.
LaPine Scientific Co. N.Y., Inc.
Lawrence Pharmaceutical, Inc.
Lederle Laboratories Division
Ledoga-Lepetit, Inc.
Leeds-Dixon Laboratories, Inc.
Leeming-Pacquin
Lehigh Valley Chemical Co.
Lemke, B. L. & Co., Inc.
Lemmon Pharmacal Co.
Leo Linden Laboratories
Lever Brothers Co.
Lif-O-Gen, Inc.
Lightfoot Company
Lilly & Co., Eli
Lily-White Sales Co., Inc.
Lincoln Laboratories, Inc.
Lloyd Brothers, Inc.
Lorvic Corporation
Luke Pharmaceutical, Inc.
Mabee-Reynard, Magnus, Inc.
MacAllister Laboratories, Inc.
Mallinckrodt Chemical Works
Marison Company
Markham Laboratories
Massengill, S. E. Co.
Matheson, Coleman & Bell
McCambridge & McCambridge Co.
McConnon & Co.
McGaw Labs, Inc.
McKesson Laboratories
McKesson & Robbins, Inc.
McNeil Laboratories, Inc.
Mead Johnson Laboratories
Medical Chemical Corp.
Medical Chemicals Corp.
Medical Gases, Inc.
Medical Supply Co.
Meer Corporation
Merck Chemical Division
Merck Sharp & Dohme
Merrell, Wm. S. Co.
Metalsalts Corporation
Microbiological Assoc., Inc.
Milan Pharmaceuticals, Inc.
Miles Chemical Co.
Millipore Filter Corp.
Mine Safety Applicances Co.
Mission Pharmacal Co.
Modern Materials Mfg. Co.
Mohawk Chemical Co., Inc.
Monsanto Company
Moore Kirk Laboratories, Inc.
Morton Chemical Co.
Moyer, J. Bird Co., Inc.
Murro Chemical Co., Inc.
Mutchler Chemical Co., Inc.
Myers Laboratories, Inc.
Myers-Carter Laboratories, Inc.
NYQ Chemical Division
Na-Spra, Inc.
National Bio Serums, Inc.
National Biological Laboratories, Inc.
National Chemical Laboratories, Penna.
National Cylinder Gas
National Drug Co.
National Package Drugs
Neoco Corporation

Nephron Company
Newport Products Co.
Nitine, Inc.
Norwich Pharmacal Co.
Novocol Chemical Mfg. Co., Inc.
Nutrilite Products, Inc.
Nutritional Biochemical Corp.
Nysco Laboratories, Inc.
Octagon Process, Inc.
Ohio Chemical & Surgical Equipment Co.
Omega Chemical Corp.
Organon, Inc.
Ortho Pharmaceutical Corp.
Orthopedic Equipment Co.
Packaging Corp. of America
Palisades Park Specialties Laboratory
Panray-Parlam Corp.
Parke, Davis & Co.
Parker, E. M. Co.
Pasadena Research Laboratories, Inc.
Pat-Ten Concentrates, Inc.
Pendergrast Chemical Co.
Penetone Company
Penick, S. B. & Co.
Pennco Distillers, Inc. of Penna.
Pennex Products Co., Inc.
Pentex Incorporated
Peroxide & Specialties Co.
Perrigo, L. Co.
Petri Wine Company
Pfanstichl Labs, Inc.
Pfeiffer Glass, Inc.
Pfizer Diagnostics
Pfizer Laboratories
Pharmachem Corporation
Pharmacia Laboratories, Inc.
Pharmetics Corporation
Pharmusa Corporation
Philips Roxane, Inc.
Phipps Products Corp.
Physicians Products Co., Inc.
Physicians & Hospitals Supply Co., Inc.
Pioneer Chemical Co., Inc.
Pioneer Laboratories
Pitman-Moore Co.
Plough, Inc.
Polak's Frutal Works, Inc.
Polichimica Spa
Premo Pharmaceutical Laboratories, Inc.
Pressed Steel Tank Co.
Private Formulae, Inc.
Proctor & Gamble Distributing Co.
Professional Pharmacal Co., Inc.
Prystan Company
Pulmosan Safety Equipment Corp.
Purdue Frederick Co.
Purecell Corporation
Purex Corporation Ltd.
Quicksilver Products, Inc.
Rabin-Winters Corp.
Rachel Laboratories
Rarisphere Corporation
Red Star Chemical Co., Inc.
Reed Products Co.
Reed & Carnrick
Republic Chemical Corp.
Requa Manufacturing Co.
Research Pharmacal Laboratory, Inc.
Rexall Drug Company
Rhodia, Inc.

Riker Laboratories
Riverton Laboratories, Inc.
Robins, A. H. Co., Inc.
Roboz Surgical Instrument Co.
Roche Laboratories
Rockland Dentil Co., Inc.
Rodana Research Corp.
Roerig, J. B. & Co.
Roselawn Laboratories, Inc.
Rowell Laboratories, Inc.
Rozer, William H., Inc.
Ryland-Johnson Co., Inc.
Salvental Chemical Products, Inc.
Salzman, Elias
Sandoz, Inc.
Savoy Drug & Chemical Co.
Schaefer, Inc.
Scherer, R. P. Spa
Schering Corporation
Schieffelin & Co.
Schimmel Co., Inc.
Scholl Mfg. Co., Inc.
Scholle Chemical Corp.
Scientific Instrument Co., Inc.
Scot Tussin Pharmacal Co., Inc.
Seaboard Mfg. Laboratories, Inc.
Searle, G. D. & Co.
Seaway Pharmacal Corp.
Sheffield Chemical Co., Inc.
Sheldon Labs, Inc.
Shell Chemical Corp.
Sherman Laboratories
Shuptrine Co.
Sinclair & Valentine Co.
Smith Kline & French Laboratories
Smith, Miller & Patch, Inc.
Sonneborn Chemical & Refining Co.
Sonorol Laboratories
Southland Industrial Products Co.
Specific Serums
Spectra Biologicals, Inc.
Spectronics Corp.
Spirt & Company, Inc.
Squibb, E. R. & Sons
Stahl Soap Co.
Standard Air Co. of N. J.
Standard Pharmacal Co.
Standard Safety Equipment Co.
Standard Scientific Supply Co.
Standard X-ray Co.
Stanley, John T. Co., Inc.
Stanley Drug Products, Inc.
Stansi Scientific Co.
Stayner Corporation
Steifel Laboratories
Stein, Hall & Co., Inc.
Sterling Drug, Inc.
Stiefel Laboratories, Inc.
Stock & Spanier, Inc.
Strasenburgh Laboratories
Strong Cobb Arner, Inc.
Stuart-Chase Corporation
Stuart Company, The
Success Chemical Co., Inc.
Summers Laboratories, Inc.
Sunlight Chemical Corp.
Swift & Co.
Sylvana Company
Syntex Laboratories, Inc.
Taylor Pharmacal Co.
Taylor, W. A. & Co.
Tenant Development Corp.
Terrell Supply Co.
Texas Pharmacal Co.
Torch Laboratories, Inc.
Travenol Laboratories, Inc.
Trio Chemical Works, Inc.

Tumbler Laboratories, Inc.
Twenty-one Brands, Inc.
Uhe, George Co., Inc.
Uni-Tech Chemical Mfg. Co.
Union Carbide Chemicals Co.
United Distillers Products Corp.
U. S. Industrial Chemicals Co.
U. S. Safety Service Co.
U. S. Vitamin & Pharmaceutical Corp.
Upjohn Company
Van Waters & Rogers, Inc.
Vaponefrin Co.
Vaughn, Inc.
Vestal Laboratories
Vi-Jon Laboratories, Inc.
Vineland Laboratories, Inc.
Vitamins, Inc.
Vitamix Pharmaceuticals, Inc.
Vitarine Co., Inc.
Wallace & Tiernan, Inc.
Wallace Laboratories
Warner-Chilcott Laboratories
Warren-Teed Products Co.
Washine Chemical Corp.
Webster, William A. Co.
West Chemical Products, Inc.
West Wholesale Drug Co.
West-ward Pharmaceuticals, Inc.
Westwood Pharmaceuticals
Wetheimer, L. E., Inc.
White Laboratories, Inc.
Whitehall Laboratories
Whorton Pharmacal Co., Inc.
Will Scientific of New York
Williams Brown-Warle, Inc.
Wilson Laboratories
Wood Ridge Chemical Corp.
WTS Pharmacroft
Xttrium Laboratories, Inc.
Yaron Laboratories, Inc.
Yates Manufacturing Co.
Yodokin, Inc.
Zemmer Co., Inc.
Zenith Laboratories, Inc.

Appendix B

Some Distributors of Generic Drugs

This list of names and addresses of distributors of generic drugs may be helpful to patients and their pharmacists. Pharmacists will know where to purchase the products of well-known brand-name manufacturers, whose names are therefore not included in this list.

Allen Pharmacal Co., Inc.
175 Pearl Street
Brooklyn, N. Y. 11201
212 UL 5-5770

American Quinine Co.
99 Hudson Street
New York, N. Y. 10013
212 CA 6-4743

Carroll Chemical Co.
2301 Hollins Street
Baltimore, Md. 21223
301 WI 5-1919

Columbia Medical Co.
38 East 19th Street
New York, N. Y. 10003
212 OR 3-7320

Consolidated Midland Corp.
15 Parkway
Katonah, N. Y.
914 CE 2-4305

Corvit Pharmaceuticals
3462 Golden Gate Way
Lafayette, Calif.
415 283-2660

Daniels, Robert, & Co., Inc.
1433-35 Boone Avenue
Bronx, N. Y. 10459
212 DA 3-2900

Horton & Converse
621 W. Pico Blvd.
Los Angeles, Calif. 90015
213 749-5161

Interstate Drug Exchange, Inc.
Skyline Drive
Plainview, L.I., N. Y. 11803
516 WE 8-9220

Kasar Laboratories
7313 N. Harlem Avenue
Niles, Ill.
312 775-7155 (Chicago)
647-8197

Lannett Company, Inc.
9000 State Road
Philadelphia, Penn. 19136
215 DE 3-9000

Panray Division
(Ormont Drug & Chemical Co.)
223 S. Dean Street
Englewood, N.J. 07631
201 567-0820
212 RA 1-2100 (N.Y.C.)

Penhurst Pharmacal Co.
315 E. Hunting Park Avenue
Philadelphia, Penn. 19124
215 GA 3-2200

Pennex Products Co., Inc.
Eastern Ave. at Pennex Drive
Verona, Penn.
412 362-5650

Raway Pharmacal Co.
2571 Atlantic Avenue
Brooklyn, N. Y. 11207
212 HY 8-7829

Rondex Laboratories, Inc.
68 Sixty-Ninth Street
Guttenberg, N. J.
201 868-5400 (N.J.)
212 LW 4-0913 (N.Y.)

Stanlabs, Inc.
(Division of Sperti Drug)
232 S.E. Oak Street
Portland, Oregon 97208
503 234-0432

Stayner Corporation
2531 Ninth Street
Berkeley, Calif. 94710
415 843-9100

Supreme Pharmaceutical Co., Inc.
354 Mercer Street
Jersey City 2, N.J.
201 432-3900

Towne, Paulsen & Co.
140 E. Duarte Road
Monrovia, Calif. 91016
213 681-6219

Vita-Fore Products Co., Inc.
95-07 98th Street
Ozone Park, N. Y.
212 VI 9-6293-4

Vitarine Co., Inc.
(Division of West Chemical
Products, Inc.)
227-15 N. Condit Avenue
Springfield Gardens, N.Y. 11413
212 AR 6-8600

West-ward Pharmaceuticals, Inc.
745 Eagle Avenue
Bronx, N. Y. 10456
212 LU 5-7777

Index

E

F

O

P

Q

T

U

V

W